William F. Haynes Jr., MD, FACC
Geffrey B. Kelly, STD, LLD

Is There a God in Health Care?
Toward a New Spirituality of Medicine

Pre-publication
REVIEWS,
COMMENTARIES,
EVALUATIONS . . .

"This book is full of powerful, fascinating stories from a cardiologist's medical practice. Here is evidence from clinical practice that prayer and faith make a difference in people's lives when they are sick. What is unique about this book is that a theologian also gives his perspective and interpretation of each case, providing a blend of both the scientific medical and deeply spiritual. Get ready to become both informed and inspired by this beautifully done book."

Harold G. Koenig, MD
*Professor of Psychiatry
and Behavioral Sciences;
Director, Center for the Study of Religion,
Spirituality, and Health,
Duke University Medical Center*

"The strength of this book lies in the obvious commitment of the authors both to its message, i.e., spirituality and prayer form the core of healing, and the truth that medicine and religion can walk hand-in-hand to bring healing to those who are sick and suffering. The answer to the initial question, whether 'there is a God in health care,' is never in doubt; the authors make their perspective known at the outset. Prayer forms a major part of their answer, but the importance of discernment as to when prayer is appropriate and welcome is also emphasized. This book is less a theological treatise than first-person accounts of God's healing in various people's lives. It provides an important example of the needed conversations between medicine and religion and how God can work through both of them."

Abigail Rian Evans, PhD, LHD, MDiv
*Professor of Practical Theology,
Princeton Theological Seminary;
Adjunct Professor of Medicine,
Robert Wood Johnson Medical School*

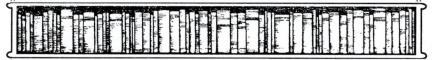

More pre-publication
REVIEWS, COMMENTARIES, EVALUATIONS . . .

"This book is a reader's delight into a journey of profound faith and unity. It presents itself in the coordination and unification of a medical doctor and a theologian. The authors offer a scholastic understanding of holistic healing combined with the power of healing prayer embedding itself into God's gift to us, that is, the Divine Physician, the Lord Jesus. One who reads these pages of a journey from human pain to the divine touch of the Healing Christ will experience a tremendous increase of hope and faith and an inspiration to anyone suffering physical, emotional, or spiritual pain. This uplifting and powerful book on medicine and prayer will serve the readers as an authentically uplifting and powerful resource. It definitely renews the broken humanity into faith in a God of wonder and might, a healing, loving Lord who continues to work wonders among people everywhere."

Rev. Ralph A. DiOrio
Director,
Apostolate of Divine Mercy and Healing,
Worcester, MA

"William F. Haynes and Geffrey B. Kelly have produced an important book that records the significant interface between religion and health care. At a time of dramatic change in the public's desire, the world over, to find works on the role of spirituality in health care, this book has a definite impact. Haynes and Kelly provide us with in-depth comment upon religion's role in health care, its supportive value in discussion of disease and preparation for end-of-life events. This book offers a comprehensive review of the subject and is, therefore, of great value in guiding health professionals, clergy, scholars, and patients as they confront this subject. It is a seminal source and reference work for all aspects of health care."

Stanley S. Bergen Jr., MD
President Emeritus,
University of Medicine and Dentistry
of New Jersey; Former Chair,
The Hastings Center

The Haworth Pastoral Press®
An Imprint of The Haworth Press, Inc.
New York • London • Oxford

NOTES FOR PROFESSIONAL LIBRARIANS AND LIBRARY USERS

This is an original book title published by The Haworth Pastoral Press®, an imprint of The Haworth Press, Inc. Unless otherwise noted in specific chapters with attribution, materials in this book have not been previously published elsewhere in any format or language.

CONSERVATION AND PRESERVATION NOTES

All books published by The Haworth Press, Inc., and its imprints are printed on certified pH neutral, acid-free book grade paper. This paper meets the minimum requirements of American National Standard for Information Sciences-Permanence of Paper for Printed Material, ANSI Z39.48-1984.

DIGITAL OBJECT IDENTIFIER (DOI) LINKING

The Haworth Press is participating in reference linking for elements of our original books. (For more information on reference linking initiatives, please consult the CrossRef Web site at www.crossref.org.) When citing an element of this book such as a chapter, include the element's Digital Object Identifier (DOI) as the last item of the reference. A Digital Object Identifier is a persistent, authoritative, and unique identifier that a publisher assigns to each element of a book. Because of its persistence, DOIs will enable The Haworth Press and other publishers to link to the element referenced, and the link will not break over time. This will be a great resource in scholarly research.

Is There a God in Health Care?
Toward a New Spirituality of Medicine

THE HAWORTH PASTORAL PRESS®
Religion and Mental Health
Harold G. Koenig, MD
Senior Editor

A Theology of God-Talk: The Language of the Heart by J. Timothy Allen

A Practical Guide to Hospital Ministry: Healing Ways by Junietta B. McCall

Pastoral Care for Post-Traumatic Stress Disorder: Healing the Shattered Soul by Daléne Fuller Rogers

Integrating Spirit and Psyche: Using Women's Narratives in Psychotherapy by Mary Pat Henehan

Chronic Pain: Biomedical and Spiritual Approaches by Harold G. Koenig

Spirituality in Pastoral Counseling and the Community Helping Professions by Charles Topper

Parish Nursing: A Handbook for the New Millennium edited by Sybil D. Smith

Mental Illness and Psychiatric Treatment: A Guide for Pastoral Counselors by Gregory B. Collins and Thomas Culbertson

The Power of Spirituality in Therapy: Integrating Spiritual and Religious Beliefs in Mental Health Practice by Peter A. Kahle and John M. Robbins

Bereavement Counseling: Pastoral Care for Complicated Grieving by Junietta Baker McCall

Biblical Stories for Psychotherapy and Counseling: A Sourcebook by Matthew B. Schwartz and Kalman J. Kaplan

A Christian Approach to Overcoming Disability: A Doctor's Story by Elaine Leong Eng

Faith, Medicine, and Science: A Festschrift in Honor of Dr. David B. Larson edited by Jeff Levin and Harold G. Koenig

Encyclopedia of Ageism by Erdman Palmore, Laurence Branch, and Diana Harris

Dealing with the Psychological and Spiritual Aspects of Menopause: Finding Hope in the Midlife by Dana E. King, Melissa H. Hunter, and Jerri R. Harris

Spirituality and Mental Health: Clinical Applications by Gary W. Hartz

Dying Declarations: Notes from a Hospice Volunteer by David B. Resnik

Maltreatment of Patients in Nursing Homes: There Is No Safe Place by Diana K. Harris and Michael L. Benson

Is There a God in Health Care? Toward a New Spirituality of Medicine by William F. Haynes and Geffrey B. Kelly

Guide to Ministering to Alzheimer's Patients and Their Families by Patricia A. Otwell

The Unwanted Gift of Grief: A Ministry Approach by Tim P. Van Duivendyk

The Treatment of Bipolar Disorder in Pastoral Counseling: Community and Silence edited by David Welton

Is There a God in Health Care?
Toward a New Spirituality of Medicine

William F. Haynes Jr., MD, FACC
Geffrey B. Kelly, STD, LLD

The Haworth Pastoral Press®
An Imprint of The Haworth Press, Inc.
New York • London • Oxford

For more information on this book or to order, visit
http://www.haworthpress.com/store/product.asp?sku=5554

or call 1-800-HAWORTH (800-429-6784) in the United States and Canada
or (607) 722-5857 outside the United States and Canada

or contact orders@HaworthPress.com

Published by

The Haworth Pastoral Press®, an imprint of The Haworth Press, Inc., 10 Alice Street, Binghamton, NY 13904-1580.

Quotation from *Daily Word* in Chapter 1 is reprinted with permission of Unity, Publisher of *Daily Word* magazine.

PUBLISHER'S NOTE

The development, preparation, and publication of this work has been undertaken with great care. However, the Publisher, employees, editors, and agents of The Haworth Press are not responsible for any errors contained herein or for the consequences that may ensue from use of materials or information contained in this work. The Haworth Press is committed to the dissemination of ideas and information contained in this work. The Haworth Press is committed to the dissemination of ideas and information according to the highest standards of intellectual freedom and the free exchange of ideas. Statements made and opinions expressed in this publication do not necessarily reflect the views of the Publisher, Directors, management, or staff of The Haworth Press, Inc., or an endorsement by them.

Identities and circumstances of some individuals discussed in this book have been changed to protect confidentiality.

Cover design by Jennifer M. Gaska.

Library of Congress Cataloging-in-Publication Data

Haynes, William F.
    Is there a God in health care? : toward a new spirituality of medicine / William F. Haynes Jr., Geffrey B. Kelly.
        p. cm.
    Includes bibliographical references and index.
    ISBN-13: 978-0-7890-2866-2 (hard : alk. paper)
    ISBN-10: 0-7890-2866-2 (hard : alk. paper)
    ISBN-13: 978-0-7890-2867-9 (soft : alk. paper)
    ISBN-10: 0-7890-2867-0 (soft : alk. paper)
    1. Medical ethics. 2. Health—Religious aspects. 3. Spirituality. 4. Religion and medicine.
I. Kelly, Geffrey B. II. Title.
    [DNLM: 1. Christianity. 2. Religion and Medicine. 3. Delivery of Health Care—methods.
4. Faith Healing—methods. 5. Pastoral Care—methods. W 61 H424i 2006]
    R725.55.H39 2006
    201.7621—dc22
                                                                            2005024103

CONTENTS

ABOUT THE AUTHORS

William F. Haynes Jr., MD, FACC, retired from office practice in 1998 after serving as a practicing internist and cardiologist for more than 40 years. He continues to teach at Robert Wood Johnson Medical School at Princeton, New Jersey, and is past President of the Cardiology Associates of Princeton. He is the author of *A Physician's Witness to the Power of Shared Prayer* and *Minding the Whole Person: Cultivating a Healthy Lifestyle from Youth Through the Senior Years.*

Geffrey B. Kelly, STD, LLD, is Chairperson of the Department of Religion at La Salle University in Philadelphia. He has published ten books in the fields of theology, spirituality, and ethics, including *Liberating Faith, A Testament to Freedom,* and *The Cost of Moral Leadership.* Dr. Kelly served two terms as President of the International Bonhoeffer Society, English Language Section, and is Founding Director of the Lasallian Leadership Institute.

Is There a God in Health Care?
© 2006 by The Haworth Press, Inc. All rights reserved.
doi:10.1300/5554_a

Foreword

The Firm Ground
on Which We Stand

It must strike readers as odd that a physician and a theologian would
write a book together about anything (except, perhaps, a mutual hobby,
such as fly-fishing, irrelevant to either's profession). Theology would
seem to have nothing to contribute to medicine, and medicine nothing
to contribute to theology. The distance between medicine and religion
in contemporary consciousness has become far wider than that between independent, specialized disciplines, such as astrophysics and
medieval English literature. The gap between medicine and religion
has become a demilitarized zone, where even the courageous fear to
tread. The conflict began many centuries ago, but by the end of the
twentieth century, medicine by and large had become openly hostile toward religion, and theologians, if they did not ignore medicine, had developed the habit of repeatedly denouncing its moral shortcomings.

Bill Haynes and Geff Kelly have therefore written a book that de-
fies expectations. They go boldly where few have gone before. Not
only do they manage to write together in a nearly seamless manner
that still leaves each a distinctive voice, they pull together all kinds of
ideas that one would ordinarily think unrelated: cardiology and mysticism, Lasallian and Franciscan spirituality, science and mindful-
ness, Bonhoeffer and faith healing. The latter most intrigues me. It
seems that it should be impossible to utter the name "Dietrich
Bonhoeffer" and the phrase "faith healing" in a grammatically correct, coherent English sentence. Yet Haynes and Kelly feature both
prominently.

If there is a connection between the theology of Dietrich Bonhoeffer and the notion of faith healing, understanding that connection

Is There a God in Health Care?
© 2006 by The Haworth Press, Inc. All rights reserved.
doi:10.1300/5554_b

might provide the key for understanding all the rest. But this connection is far from obvious. There would seem to be no reasonable place from which to start. Bonhoeffer is the theologian of world engagement, the father of "religionless Christianity." One could almost not imagine a theologian less likely to attend a faith healing service. His theology is at times so *this*-wordly that one wonders if he ever thought seriously about the notion of the miraculous, never mind *what* he might have thought about it. At other times his writing is so cerebral that it would not seem that he could brook any discussion of the supernatural. As one of the authors, Geff Kelly, has written elsewhere, Bonhoeffer "spurned what he considered the misleading 'religious trappings' of Christianity. The God of extramundane solutions to life's problems, the so-called 'stopgap God' or *deus ex machina* was unreal to him."[1] Faith healing, however, would seem to be the paradigmatic *deus ex machina* event, the ultimate extramundane solution to the problem of illness. Could Bonhoeffer, or a Christian impressed by his theology, have any faith in miraculous cures? There are a few passing mentions of the words "miracle" and "miraculous" in Bonhoeffer's writings, but the prospect of a robust theology of miraculous healing seems remote. He writes,

> A few more words about "religionlessness." I expect you remember Bultmann's essay on the "demythologizing" of the New Testament? My view of it today would be, not that he went "too far," as most people thought, but that he didn't go far enough. It's not only the mythological concepts . . . but "religious" concepts generally, which are problematic. You can't, as Bultmann supposes, separate God and miracle, but you must be able to interpret and proclaim *both* in a "non-religious" sense.[2]

Despite the apparent obstacles posed by such a passage, the authors of this book hold tenaciously both to Bonhoeffer's theology and to the religious significance of faith healing. They pursue careful study of works such as *The Cost of Discipleship* and also believe in Charismatic prayer for miraculous cures. How in the world is this possible?

One might venture to say that only Christ could hold all of this together. Ewert Cousins described St. Bonaventure's Christology as a "coincidence of opposites."[3] Although religious language is often paradoxical, Cousins reads Bonaventure as claiming that Christ is the paradox of ultimate significance. In Christ are death and life, immanence and transcendence, humanity and divinity, the alpha and the omega. He is, as Bonaventure says, the "intelligible sphere whose center is everywhere, and whose circumference is nowhere."[4] Perhaps one must conclude that only such a sphere could contain both Bonhoeffer and faith healing.

True as this might be, however, such a treatment of the question would still be too facile. It sounds too "religious," in the pejorative sense in which Bonhoeffer uses the word to describe our all-too-frequent use of religious language and ritual to escape from genuine religious truth. To subsume all of life's paradoxes under Christ might tell us something about Christ, but unless one can say *how* they are subsumed under Christ, they remain paradoxical and unexplained.

Nor does it help much, in describing how contemporary theology and faith healing can be reconciled, to say simply, "It is a mystery." That is because, in a truly religious sense, the word "mystery" does not refer to an absence of explanation, an absence of knowledge, or a lacuna in our scientific account of the world. In a truly religious sense, mystery has a positive content. Mystery created the world. Mystery calls us. Mystery is at the deep center of each person. We are created in the image of that Mystery.

Whatever we know about miracles, whether the appearance of God in a burning bush or the cure of a man born blind, it is fair to say that a miracle is always an encounter with mystery. Therefore, as with "mystery," "miracle" cannot simply be a word we use to describe what we do not understand. In Bonhoeffer's words, this would be to treat God as a "stopgap." If the word "miracle" were defined as an event that cannot be explained scientifically, then the word would cease to have any meaning in medicine. Medical science understands so little that everything, even the relief of a headache by aspirin, would then be a miracle. This is because, in a strict sense, if one pursues all the relevant questions to their ends, nothing that is particular can ever be explained completely. Scientific explanation is about the universal, not the particular. Medical practice, by contrast, while scientifically informed, is always particular—*this* patient, *these* symptoms, *these* circumstances. Therefore, on principle, one can readily deduce why I can never fully understand why any medicine I prescribe does or does not cure a given patient who fits the average profile of someone for whom such a medicine is indicated. Yet this inability to offer a complete explanation surely does not mean that I am a miraculous healer. If every cure is a miracle, then no cure is a miracle.

So, if the word "miracle" is to have any meaning in our religious vocabulary, miracles must have more to do with the way we experience certain discrete events in our lives than they do with our inability to offer rational, scientific·explanations for them. Miracles are events in which mystery is made manifest to us in some new, startling, and significant way. Miracles are experiences that disclose to us our radical dependence upon a mystery that is knowable.

Events unfold in our lives. Sometimes, if we are attentive, they unfold in a way that is unexpected, erupting with abundant grace, spilling forth upon the dreary plain of our daily routine, filling us with gratitude and wonder, answering our deepest longings, and pointing out what is really and always true. A husband, given up for dead, might be extracted alive from the wreckage of an earthquake. A daughter, diagnosed before birth as profoundly retarded and a candidate for elective "termination," might be delivered from her mother's womb as a normal, bright, and healthy baby. A poor peasant might see the Mother of God, for a fleeting moment, trembling before a vision of a woman clothed with the sun.

Miracles emerge from our reflections about such events. A miracle is a judgment. In retrospect, with time, in consultation with others, we arrive at a judgment about an event that has already occurred and come to understand what it means—a miracle has occurred. Thus understood, miracles are not characterized by the scientific quantification and verification of human limitation. Of this we need no more proof. Miracles concern that which transcends our limitation—the real answer to our hearts' every prayer.

The task of theology has never been to offer general, *a priori* systems of thought from which events in God's world can be deduced. *Fides quaerens intellectum* implies, by theology's own definition, that faith comes first. Faithfulness in the way one takes up one's own life; faithfulness in the way one sees the world and holds one's place in the world; the stand of faith assumes priority of place.

And so, no one should expect that Bonhoeffer will tell us whether we should go to faith healing services. But if his theology is worth studying, it must have something to say to a sophisticated theologian who folds his dying young daughter in his arms, suffering as she is with a cancer pronounced incurable by her doctors, and walks slowly down the aisle of a church toward the altar, begging God for mercy, asking why she should suffer so, and crying out for help. In such an event, the frailty of our human creatureliness confronts the eternal mysteries of faith, hope, and love. Such a person takes full consideration of his life, of the lives of those he loves, and with due regard turns his gaze upon the whole universe before which he stands. At the center of such an event lies faith—faith in hope; faith in love; faith in the Mystery. The task of theology is not to permit or to prohibit such events, but to explain how in the world such events happen.

Is Bonfoeffer up to this task? Haynes and Kelly remind us that while he was in a Nazi prison, facing his own death, Bonhoeffer wrote the following words to his friend, Eberhard Bethge,

> It is certain that we can claim nothing for ourselves, and yet may pray for everything; it is certain that our joy is hidden in suffering, and our life in death; it is certain that in all this we are in a fellowship that sustains us. In Jesus, God has said Yes and Amen to it all, and that Yes and Amen is the firm ground on which we stand.[5]

All cures are temporary. But our deepest human urges are not. Bonhoeffer reminds us that the Amen of Christ is the only firm place wherein we can stake our claim for that which is not temporary; for that which is our birthright in the Mystery that has formed us and sustains us.

Miracles are events that disclose Christ as the author of life and announce his victory over death. Miracles teach us that Christ is the only firm ground on which we can stand, whether we are healthy or sick, rejoicing or grieving, recovering or growing worse. Whether we are patients or practitioners; insured by Medicaid or Aetna; in a fee-for-service system or a national health service; whether we live or die, we are the Lord's (Romans 14:8).

If one reads him carefully, Bonhoeffer seems to insist that both the words "God" and "miracle" will require a "religionless" interpretation if we are ever to recover a truly religious understanding of either. Haynes and Kelly offer us a glimpse into how this might be possible, through healing and faith; technology and mysticism; science and spirit; the mundane and the miraculous; medicine and theology—in the coincidence of opposites—our one firm ground—Jesus Christ.

Daniel P. Sulmasy, OFM, MD, PhD
Chair, John J. Conley Department of Ethics,
Saint Vincents Hospital and Medical Center;
Professor of Medicine and Director of the Bioethics Institute
of New York Medical College

NOTES

1. Geffrey B. Kelly, *Liberating Faith: Bonhoeffer's Message for Today* (Minneapolis: Augsburg Press, 1984), p. 131.

2. Dietrich Bonhoeffer, *Letters and Papers from Prison,* ed. Eberhard Bethge (New York: Macmillan, 1972), p. 285.

3. Ewert H. Cousins, *Bonaventure and the Coincidence of Opposites* (Chicago: Franciscan Herald Press, 1978).

4. St. Bonaventure, *Bonaventure: Selected Spiritual Writings* "The Soul's Journey into God," *(Itinerarium Mentis in Deum)* V.8, trans. Ewert H. Cousins (New York: Paulist Press, 1978), p. 100.

5. Bonhoeffer, *Letters and Papers from Prison,* p. 391.

Preface

Theologian Geff's Comments

A typical way for an Irishman such as me to evade answering a very complex question is usually: "Well, it's a long story!" I anticipate being asked how Bill and I came to write this book. How did a medical doctor come to collaborate with a theologian in an area that often leaves behind the world of the empirical and the predictable? Well, it is a long story! A short answer could be that we imagined we might be the two personae of Saint Luke who has been described in the Christian tradition as both a theologian and a physician. Whether or not he was a bona fide physician, there is no doubt that Luke, author of the third Gospel, speaks with unmatched theological eloquence of the healing presence and power of Jesus Christ. As does Luke, we too wish to share with the reader our thoughts on how prayer and the spiritual life, empowered by the continued presence of the Holy Spirit, are at the core of the healing power of God, so present in Jesus of Nazareth. We are convinced that the same power that inspirited the prophets of old, and now, in our own time, is manifested in the diverse ways in which healing takes place both within and adjacent to the practice of medicine. The invocation of that compassionate energy is sadly an untapped resource of healing in which God has gifted each one of us.

I first met Dr. Bill Haynes when he was a student in my graduate religion course on "The Healing Teaching Ministry of Jesus." I knew only that he was a recently retired cardiologist and internist who wanted to take courses in theology and spirituality in order to enrich his life beyond the practice of medicine and to fortify his credentials on spirituality and healing when lecturing in hospitals to medical students, fellow physicians, and various community groups. I never had a retired senior citizen student in my courses, and I harbored the belief that retirement years always meant a dramatic scaling down of the stressful work of a long professional career. In Bill's case, I imagined he had distanced himself from the intensity of his usual medical practice or had drastically reduced his "working" hours. Because his lovely wife, Aline, had phoned me earlier to inquire if he had been accepted into our program, I asked myself: "How old is this guy? I'll bet she's really anxious to get him out of the house." I was wrong. In the opening session of the course, I did not expect to meet in Bill a person with rather a youthful face and apparently in great physical condition, even with a young man's bounce to his step. I did not know then that he was a competitive swimmer while at Princeton University and has continued competing in that sport, ranking in the "Top Ten" in backstroke (for his age group) in the U.S. Master Swimming program. Also, he was engaged in teaching medical students in the field of cardiology and gave talks to hospitals and to various gatherings about the need for caregivers to integrate their spiritual faith into the practice of medicine. It was a lesson Bill and I had learned through painful experience.

I began my course, as I do all my courses, with introductions so my students can tell each other something of themselves to the limits of their comfort with such personal sharing. I always take the lead in this, describing in very capsule form my own life with a couple of its defining turns, my educational background, my faith, my twenty some years in religious life as a De La Salle Christian Brother, and my hopes that we would not only learn from the texts, but also learn from one another. I try to break down some of the usual reserve of students and lessen the tension of my "teacher expectations" for them. I have a reputation for taking a lighthearted, friendly approach to my courses and for having a teasing way of getting people to share not only their intellectual insights but their ideas on how to apply to real life what we are reading and analyzing.

But when Bill spoke I could see a few brows arching when he mentioned that he was a semiretired doctor anxious to enrich his understanding of faith and the spiritual life through the versatile program that La Salle University was offering. I felt flattered. Bill told the students—all younger than he—how much he had come to appreciate prayer and faith in his own medical practice. Somehow, the vibrations of the other students seemed to convey to me that this guy had to be very educated and would probably overwhelm them with his more erudite, scientific opinions on all sorts of things. If that were the case, I am sure that they were all surprised when they discovered that this

Dr. Haynes was as eager to learn as they were, and that at heart he was, and is, an unpretentious "regular guy."

Sometimes in my courses we share our own life stories at the deeper level impossible on the first evening. In courses on Jesus, that often happens in reaction to the texts under study. Students begin to express to each other how the teachings and healings of Jesus have impacted them in their various ministries. One evening we were discussing how the brokenness of heart can sadden a person's life or how an overwhelming sense of sin can lead to unexpected moments in which a person, overwhelmed with sadness and indescribable anguish, can become more open to the powerful healing presence of God. It was at this time that Bill told the class that he too had been broken into little pieces like a piece of china dropped from a tall building. The class was breathless as he described the way God had touched his life in a way totally unexpected after he had been toppled from his high perch as a very busy physician with an all encompassing career in his full possession.

I found myself identifying with Bill because I too had experienced a brokenness of heart and an intense need for the kind of healing that Bill describes in more detail in this book. Later I will share that experience with the reader in its proper context. This book began as our third course together. As he edged closer to his Master's degree in Graduate Religion from La Salle University, Bill proposed that he do an independent study on a topic of our mutual interest. I counterproposed that Bill write his third book, namely, something on spirituality in medical healing, and I would attempt to be his most critical editor and literary whip. He agreed. However, not too many pages into his "book," it became apparent that, while I liked Bill's anecdotal way of relating prayer and spirituality to the healing processes, both he and I were less than satisfied with his attempts to relate this to contemporary theology and biblical interpretation. I suggested so many rewrites that Bill challenged me to stop the flow of red ink on the material that was less in the area of his expertise and actually become a co-author of the book. I would be responsible for doing the theology and biblical analysis; he would continue to tell those fascinating stories that illustrate ways in which medical healing is enhanced when and if physicians are able to incorporate faith, prayer, and their inner spirituality into the process of healing.

As a result, Bill's independent study became much more complicated for him and more demanding on me. I told him our partnership would double his work, lengthen his paper, and add a volatile degree of difficulty when we tried to integrate our two approaches to healing. Bill would be coming from the purely scientific background of a physician, and I from the very religious background of a theologian. He was in a profession dedicated to healing various ills of patients, while I labored as a teacher to overcome intellectual ignorance and spiritual aimlessness among very typical college students. But what we had in common, our brokenness, our reliance on prayer, our personal, relational approaches to healing and teaching, and, finally, our common faith in the powers that God has implanted in our humanity, made our collaboration a pleasant one. We hope that our personal experiences in healing and teaching will help readers appreciate more deeply the power of healing that we have ourselves experienced.

Doctor Bill's Comments

I have been in the private practice of internal medicine and cardiology in Princeton, New Jersey, for the past thirty-eight years, but it has been only during the past twenty years that I have been praying with patients. My role in writing this book is to allow the book to be a source of encouragement for all caregivers regardless of their formal education. I am convinced that not only is there great power in shared prayer, but that many benefits previously unexpected can accrue not only to the patient, but to the caregiver as well. Even though much that will be said comes from the perspective of a practicing physician, this can apply to all who serve in healing ministries, be they medical personnel, theologians, or laypeople. I do not consider myself a biblical expert or a theologian, but I feel very secure having Dr. Geff Kelly add his unique perspective regarding the broad subject of healing. Geff is a well-known theologian who agreed to bail me out if I wandered too far theologically. We both share the common belief that prayer can be a powerful force in the healing process.

From the physician's point of view, I have been blessed in having witnessed the results of prayer in a wide variety of medical illnesses. We hope to meld the two vocations, modern scientific medicine with biblical-theological interpretations in a synergistic manner, into a unified approach in dealing with the many wounds and complexities of today's world. By bringing together these two vocations, linked together by a bond of compassion, the book will, we hope, be a powerful testimony for God's important role in the ministry of healing as we find ourselves living in a high-tech and increasingly secular world. In addition, those of us who profess to be Christians have been called to be disciples of Jesus Christ who prayed earnestly to his father God. Sometimes we need to be reminded that we do not have to be "certified" to pray. I mention this because doctors are very conscious about being "trained" to perform most medical services, and since few are ordained, they tend to be reticent in employing prayer as an adjunct to good medical practice.

During my first twenty years of practice, I was neither open nor bold enough to pray with patients. In my opinion, we were trained as action-oriented clinicians, and we entered into the practice of medicine with a total lack of training in things spiritual. At least so it was in my case. If someone was in need of an inner healing due to a broken relationship, a feeling of rejection, some unresolved guilt, or even a feeling of despair, I would prescribe valium, give a pat on the back, or a referral to a psychiatrist; I was too zipped-up and encased in a brick wall to do otherwise. Patients who were obviously in need of prayer and emotional support caused me to feel uneasy and awkward. I fenced myself off from addressing those issues. Treating pneumonia or a heart attack was far easier for me.

The second half of my career has been much different in many ways. My own loss (a totally unwanted divorce), and its associated pain in 1980, was the necessary jump-start for changing my life's direction and beginning a life of daily prayer. Strangely enough, once I had become "broken," I then subsequently became "open" to God's healing presence. It was the time for a profound spiritual journey to unfold. I sensed a new and compelling approach to medical practice—a blending of soul and science. I will elaborate on this in more detail later, but a verse from Psalm 51 seemed very pertinent that time: "Let me hear joy and gladness; let the bones that you have crushed rejoice" (Psalm 51:8).

Having experienced the power of prayer in my own life—the role it played in my own inner healing, then it seemed logical to consider using prayer with patients. Soon after, I began to incorporate prayer into my daily routine as a physician. I witnessed how God answered my prayers, deepened my own faith, brought great joy to me personally, and radically enhanced my options in medical practice. I also realized that optimum care required treating the "whole person"—mind, body, and spirit. I likened this to a three-legged stool; unless all three legs were in order, the stool would not function as it should. The "spiritual" leg had never been mentioned during our medical school and postgraduate training, and with few exceptions, this is the rule today. I hope that this book will help others bring spirituality and prayer into the various ministries both medical and spiritual that form the healing professions.

My first class with Professor Geff Kelly, in studying the teaching, healing ministry of Jesus, made me realize that he too had been broken, a fact that he shared with us during our first session. I remember him saying that at one time he was basking in great success professionally: writing books, teaching, giving retreats, a recipient of numerous awards, traveling all over the country and abroad. He remarked, "I thought I was another Henri Nouwen until I held my young daughter in my arms in an emergency room at Children's Hospital, knowing she was dying from a brain tumor." He continued, "You know what? I realized then that all my accomplishments were nothing!"

Geff's vulnerability has transformed his life. Today, he is one of the most sought-after and gifted professors on the faculty. His love for God and his church is apparent to all of his students. Through the prayers of many people and the help of multiple medical and surgical procedures, his daughter is alive fifteen years later. Her lively persona far outshines the relatively modest neurological impairments that remain. She remains constantly bathed in prayers by family, friends, and students. That she is still alive is a tribute to the faith and prayers that have sustained her and promoted the healing that has renewed both her life and Geff's. I am glad that Geff tells Susan's story in this book.

Our Faith and Spiritual Perspective in the Ministry of Health Care

We acknowledge that our reflections in this book on the ministry of health care are fundamentally rooted in our personal Christian faith and religious background. At the same time we do not wish in any way to disparage other religions or other denominations that have been outstanding in their contributions to the ministry of health care. We count among our esteemed colleagues in health care representatives of nearly every religion as well as the different denominations within those religions. We believe that there is in all world religions, and even among humanist nonbelievers, an innate goodness and compassion. Whatever the country or religions involved, these health care-givers are doing battle courageously and effectively against the forces destructive of human life around the globe. We concede upfront the limitations of our personal faith and religious experience. We are only conscious of lighting one candle to chase away some of the darkness that threatens to overwhelm the ministry of health care. We hope that those of other faiths, as well as nonbelievers, can find in these pages a source of hope and an encouragement in their varied work as health care providers. Our dream is that this book could perhaps serve as a resource for an ecumenical dialogue with focus on how each of our respective religions and their faithful understand and carry out this important ministry.

Although at times we use *spirituality* and *faith* interchangeably, by spirituality we mean the yearning or deep hunger within us as human beings in our search for the "something more" or the "transcending" aspect of our lives. Spirituality is, as the word implies, how we relate to and are formed by God's Spirit into the better human beings we are called by God to be. This is the story of how God's Spirit encounters and transforms us into loving, compassionate, caring people. In our Christian perspective we can speak of how God's Spirit may form us into the likeness of Jesus Christ. Our spirituality allows us to experience that which is most fulfilling in human existence, to enter into communion with God's world, and thus become channels of love, community, healing, and peace for those who are part of our own community and the wider world.

How we express this relationship leads us to enter into communities of faith in which we, together with others of a like mind and belief, honor God and serve one another. Prayer is the way we commune with God in our life's journey. Prayer is a privileged mode of our being with God, often in the deepest recesses of our hearts, in order to experience not only the love and tenderness of God but also to listen to the words that God speaks to us to restore our energies, to console us, and to free us up to serve others. In prayer we can address our needs and problems to a Father who cares for us. Likewise, in prayer we can experience in ourselves and extend to others the healing and peace that we acknowledge as God's beneficent outreach to a troubled creation. It can be both communal and individual. It can take on many forms. Realizing that there is no absolute formula for or style of prayer, we decided to approach this phenomenon by describing several paths in prayer with an emphasis on the personal way in which God began and nurtured in us a love for prayer and enabled us to pray in the healing process in which we are involved.

To the extent that we have completed this book with any success in helping others in the healing professions, we are indebted to several people. We acknowledge, first of all, the support of our families who encouraged us to stay with the project because the book promised to be of great help to both those who are health caregivers and those who are in need of help in their various illnesses to which humans are subject. We are grateful, too, to our colleagues at Princeton and La Salle University, the medical professionals and the bioethicists who have urged us to complete the book as a well-needed service in all the fields connected with the practice of medicine. We hope that this book will help health care providers everywhere to bring their spirituality and prayer life into the various divisions of works of healing that comprise the ministry of health care. We thank Dennis Feltwell, Neil Dougherty, and Denny Whalen for their meticulous reading of the original manuscript. We are likewise grateful to Yvonne Macolly, secretary to the Department of Religion at La Salle University, for her patience in helping us prepare the typescript for submission. We acknowledge, too, the helpful suggestions of editors Dawn Krisko and Peg Marr at The Haworth Press. We are especially grateful to Doctor Daniel P. Sulmasy, who is both a medical doctor and a Franciscan Brother, for his thought-provoking Foreword. From the very beginning of this book, Dr. Sulmasy's experiential insights help the reader to overcome the seeming disparity between the scientific-medical and the spiritual in the practice of health care. Finally we are grateful to our wives, Aline Linehan Haynes and Joan Wingert Kelly, for their endless patience in freeing us for the time we needed to write and revise the text and their encouragement as this book began its gestation in places as far apart as Princeton and Philadelphia, Bill's medical practice, and the religion department's lounge at La Salle University.

Chapter 1

The Power of Prayer
in the Health Care Ministries

REFLECTIONS

Doctor Bill

Imagine a practice where the first words spoken by a patient upon entering my office for a routine visit are: "Don't forget, before I leave we have to pray together." This comes as a joy for me and quite a turnaround from the first half of my professional career! This is not the case for every patient, but each time it occurs is very special to me. Patients today are increasingly more open to prayers—they have even *requested* them. But if I discern that a particular patient does not want an audible prayer or even the hint of prayers on his or her behalf, I then pray for that individual silently, knowing that even silent prayers can be heartfelt and a genuine source of God's gracious blessings.

Whenever an individual prays with another, a great amount of love is expressed. One who prays must care enough to take time to be present, to listen, even to lay hands in prayer on the other person, and to ask God to use him or her as a channel of healing. This is a form of love in action. When the prayer is direct, to the point, and asks God's help for a specific condition or illness, this is what I call a *prayer of intercession*. At times, a prayer of affirmation may be even stronger and more powerful because of the faith it demands, since we are thanking God for a healing we presume is already underway.

Unless otherwise noted, Bible verses quoted in this book are from the New Revised Standard Version (NRSV).

Regardless of the form of prayer used, a bond is formed, a special connection, between the people involved. Praying *with* someone can have a healing quality greater than praying *for* someone. It develops an authentic spiritual relationship. In my view, it is more powerful than saying, "I'll pray for you in church" or "I'll have my prayer group put your name on our list."

The reminder of our obligation to pray together came from the milkman who used to drive up from Delaware to Princeton for his blood pressure and diabetes checkup every four months. Our visits ended with prayers for each other and thanks to God for looking after each of us. We had more than a doctor-patient relationship. We were spiritual friends. We would catch up with each other to see what God had been doing with our lives. Were our prayers being answered? Were more prayers needed for a special situation? Had there been some unexpected blessings that we could rejoice about? No matter what the prayer agenda is, by the end of each visit we both felt uplifted and reassured of God's never-ending presence and help.

The practice of prayer with and for our patients can be of immense help during the decision-making process when there is a lot of confusion and little time for what could be a life or death judgment. One incident that I will never forget helped me realize that sometimes the best we can do is to turn the problem immediately over to God.

I arrived on the medical floor of the hospital one weekday morning and was greeted by several nurses, the night shift going off and the day shift about to start. They were concerned about Helen, a forty-year-old patient, who had been disturbing everyone all night by crying out, shouting, jumping out of bed, lying on the floor, and even banging her head on the floor. She was also being abusive to the nursing staff and house officers. She had been given a sedative for agitation without effect. I had known Helen for a long time. She had survived many years of torment as she struggled with both alcohol and drug abuse. In recent years, she seemed to be doing much better. We had even prayed together from time to time, giving thanks for all the good things that were happening in her life. I looked on her as a living example of God's grace.

On this morning, however, she was apparently suffering a severe migraine attack. I prayed for the Spirit to speak through me as I hurried to her room. The nursing supervisor and a number of patients were all watching to see the fireworks. I felt that I was in the spotlight and besieged by everyone on the floor to "do something"—to not only correct the condition immediately, but to do so to everyone's satisfaction. After I helped Helen back to bed and held her hand, we prayed together for God to come into her heart and give her peace and love. As I sat with her, I could see her become more relaxed and peaceful. She eventually quieted down and went to sleep. Helen was a model patient for the remaining three days of her hospital stay. Her "seizure" was largely due to the migraine attack accompanied by agitation and hyperventilation. But the Lord brought her peace using me as an instrument of caring. When the others asked me what happened, I smiled and said simply, "We prayed together," and walked away. But something did happen. In opening my mind and heart to the Holy Spirit, I believe that I was led to choose the words that would soothe and comfort most. I am convinced that the Holy Spirit will guide our words and actions as long as we remain open to this source of God's own empowerment in our ministry of health care.[1]

The work of healing our ills, whether they be physical, spiritual, or emotional, takes place primarily in the spiritual, relationship in faith with which God has gifted us if we choose to accept it. A genuine spirituality inspired by faith can infuse a dynamic power into today's health care ministries. Faith and prayer have an enormous impact on physical, spiritual, and emotional wellness. Understanding how one's spirituality can help in providing health care requires the human qualities of faith, hope, and love, which are pure gifts on God's part, eliciting in turn our trust in what God's presence and healing power can accomplish in our daily lives. Accepting these gifts and entering into a personal relationship with God is shown in our becoming more loving and compassionate in dealings with others and continuing to trust in God's goodness and providential care present within us. At times, this faith has taken the form of a recognition that God can and does indeed work wonders through the dedicated work of those involved in health care at every level of patient need and a willingness to work with God in the care of those confided to our care.

Research suggests that spirituality and prayer play a more vital role in the healing process than was formerly thought when technology dominated the medical profession. In my experience, the impetus to a vital patient–physician bond can only be enhanced through prayer. At this time of high-tech bioengineering, HMOs (health maintenance organizations), malpractice suits, medical denials, and unhappy, uninsured, and underinsured patients, hasty and often impersonal care, overwhelming paperwork, it is no wonder there is a great need for a caregiver's attentive ear—and, for patients, there is a need to trust their caregivers in times of illness.

Biotechnology is wonderful, but it must not permanently distance physicians from their patients. We must preserve the time-tested, "hands-on" care as well. Physical examinations force doctors to touch their patients and help to create a physical bond which is recognized to be an important factor in the art of healing.[2] The physical exam, however, should not be limited to such contact only during episodes of debilitating illness. Doctors should get to know their patients while they enjoy full health. Some doctors' offices prefer using a "Medical History Form" whereby health questions are asked of the patient. The individual then checks the appropriate box, allowing a "yes" or a "no." This approach may save the physician time, but it can also remove the eye contact, body language, and the spontaneity vital to establishing and sustaining a good doctor-patient relationship.

In prayer together, the doctor and the patient not only experience a more joyful and trusting relationship, but they also achieve a better patient compliance: keeping appointments, taking medications, and making necessary lifestyle changes. Last but not least, by praying for each other's concerns and needs, both parties can receive a gift of inner peace. The benefits of this kind of relationship when compared to what has been experienced in practices of medicine limited to the purely scientific, technological, and pharmacological have no limits. Of course, it is presupposed that the doctor and the patient both believe in a God who has the compassion and the power to heal our ills.

Pollsters such as George Gallup and Andrew Greeley have found that over 90 percent of Americans believe in God. A *Newsweek* poll revealed that 87 percent of Americans believe that God answers prayers.[3] This is quite striking when one considers the great religious diversity present in this country. Equally remarkable is that, in our secular society, which worships the idols of the "self" and material success, we can find the time, space, and even the need to worship God. Today there seems to be an awakening, a revival, a renewal of faith, as many successful individuals apparently blessed with worldly goods, are noticing "something missing" in life—a yearning for a deeper meaning beyond the totems of their material success.

Perhaps there is a realization that inner peace comes from living our faith in God rather than placing our faith in the "self" or material things. Caregivers, in their daily profession of helping others, soon realize that even prosperity does not insulate the patient from life's hurts. This trend is further evidenced by the increasing number of publications on spirituality that appear each year in the media. Books about faith are among the top sellers. It seems as if God has been invited to "come out of the closet." The public is less apprehensive about discussing issues of faith, spirituality, and healing. Those in need are more and more open to healing prayers, and this cuts across all social barriers. The physician who prays, therefore, can have two roles: the traditional one dealing with medical care, and the spiritual one. This will be illustrated in actual cases later on in this book.

The challenge to health care workers is that they must also be humble, even willing, when appropriate, to share some of their own personal difficulties and woundedness. When done with discretion, this openness can be a powerful instrument of healing for the suffering patient. Genuine, heartfelt prayer shows an attitude of caring, and this caring in turn can foster healing. The following words from the *Daily Word* nicely reinforced this for me: "Any care that we give one member of the family of God surely must honor God and the whole family of God. The caregivers of the world give from the Spirit of God within them. We are all caregivers."[4] The human touch during prayer adds another dimension of caring, when done with appropriate reverence. Sometimes a gentle touch can be by itself a prayer while no words need be spoken.

A Note of Caution

When dealing with the subject of prayer and healing, we cannot overstate the need for discernment, since we never want to intrude on anyone's spiritual privacy. This could be very offensive. But in health care, once we detect that a person is open to prayer, and after asking permission, we can then proceed. If the patient is not open to audible prayer, we can still intercede quietly. Remember that in prayer the caregiver becomes only a channel for God's spirit to effect the petitioned healing. We may become the instruments of what God accomplishes. God is the healer, not we humans. The basis for successful prayer for both the one who prays and the one who is prayed for, is to have the necessary faith that God is present and answers prayers. The answer to a particular prayer may take time and may be answered in a way different from what was expected.

Since we believe the Lord is involved in all healing, whether physical, emotional, or spiritual, we are also convinced that any amelioration of a patient's condition will be at God's own timing and outcome, not ours. We must learn to trust that God has a special plan for each of us. "What do you think God's plan is for *you*?" It is likely none of us will ever know God's designs on us in any great detail, if we do not take the time to listen to God's divine guidance on a daily basis. God always beckons us—but are we listening? Over time we may become similar to the psalmist who reiterates God's constant presence: "but God has surely listened and heard my voice in prayer. Praise be to God, who has not rejected my prayer or withheld his love from me!" (Psalm 66:19-20).

In some illnesses, an answer to a given prayer may be a *healing*—but not necessarily a *cure*. This has to be recognized when praying for the terminally ill. The dying person can receive *spiritual healings* such as decreased pain, reconciliation with family members or friends, decreased anxiety, or better sleep patterns. Likewise, *physical healings* may include loss of a rash, healing of a skin ulcer, decreased fever, improved appetite, and perhaps a decrease in side effects from medications. These healings testify to God's presence and grace. God is ever-faithful, and prayers will be heard—although not always with the outcome we request! In a time of trial and suffering, we can take some comfort in the knowledge that we are not suffering alone; God suffers with us.

Theologian Geff

Bill's last comment reminds me of what Dietrich Bonhoeffer had written from prison before his execution: "Only a suffering God can help us."[5] Bill's words of caution about the difference between a physical cure and a healing are important here for two reasons. First, it is easy for successful physicians who have added prayer for the patient to their repertoire in restoring a patient to good health to be deluded that the power is all theirs. This healing power is not a personal weapon against disease or an efficient talisman to ward off death and add to the glamour of a physician's reputation. Rather, it is the power of God's spirit flowing through the physician, the nurse, the hospice care provider, and others involved in the healing ministries. We believe that God is the source of all healing even as that power is extended to those human instruments who become God's access to people in their times of physical, spiritual, and emotional distress.

And this is related to the second caution: spiritual, psychological, and, at times, even a bodily healing is different from a "cure." The story of Dr. Alexis Carrel provides a good illustration of this distinction. He went to Lourdes as a cynical agnostic in order, as a scientist, to disprove the claims of the nature-defying wonders that were taking place among several "hopeless" people seeking miraculous cures. He came away a believer, not because of any spectacular cure he had witnessed, but because of the faith he saw in the faces of those whose petitions for their loved ones were *not answered* with a dramatic cure. What he witnessed, instead, was the even more "miraculous" healing of hearts broken as the lives of their loved ones continued to slip away and diseases continued to run their natural course. Their resignation to the inevitable, their continued blessing of God, their conviction that God did, indeed, continue to care for them, their confession of faith in God's promise of life after this life—these were the unspectacular, inner wonders that moved the agnostic physician to become a person of deep and lasting faith.[6]

As Bill mentioned, the distinction between spiritual *healings* and physical *cures* is important, lest one distort the meaning of faith and turn prayers for the terminally ill into an occasion to doubt the power of prayer and the goodness of God in the midst of life's calamitous turns and chaotic unpredictability. The prayer that Bill cites is a prayer of supreme confidence. Yet the question of what the psalmist was praying for is left unanswered. And, lingering on the minds of some at least, may be the number of times when they are unable to declare with the psalmist that God "has not rejected my prayer." The issue of how God answers prayers is alluded to here but will be addressed by us at greater length in another context. Prayers for the terminally ill and prayers in general can become, in effect, an emotional challenge to belief in the goodness and power of God.

Spiritual and emotional healing is, indeed, different from a physical cure or complete recovery from a bodily illness. When given a choice, few people suffering from both moral guilt and some form of paralysis would rather have their sins forgiven and guilt alleviated than be given the gift of walking again. Yet, the priority of forgiveness over recovery from the physical ailment of paralysis seems to be the very point of the paralytic's cure in Mark 2:1-12. When the paralytic is lowered through the roof of the house where Jesus is teaching and presented before him, Jesus says: "Your sins are forgiven." It would be a safe wager that those words were not exactly what the paralytic or his friends wanted to hear. Yet, in Jesus' view, it was more important to be reconciled to God and enjoy peace of soul than to be able to walk of one's own accord. Forgiveness, or reconciliation, has priority.

Some critics of the text argue that the paralysis from which the man suffered was obviously psychosomatic and had moral guilt as its cause, hence Jesus' words of forgiveness were a psychological uplift as a prelude to the more dramatic physical miracle.[7] Others see this solely as Jesus' setting the stage for a theatrical display of his power to heal the sick and confound his enemies. Still others see this as Mark's attempt to place Jesus on a level with God who, in the orthodox Jewish theology extant at the time, alone had the power to forgive sins. Certainly one could make a case for a little bit of all these analyses. However, the main point of the Markan story might still be missed. Jesus came to bring peace on earth, a peace that, as he said at the Last Supper, the world cannot give (see John 14:27). To be reconciled with God, with one another, and oneself, would be the more powerful wonder in Jesus' ability to heal the wounds of both soul and body. In other words, Jesus' primary mission was *not to work miracles.* The miracles were nothing more than attestations of Jesus primary intent to bring new life to sinners.

This power is a gift that Jesus told his followers they could exercise. They were to forgive sins in his name, forgiving even their enemies or executioners, thereby, giving an example of just how far-reaching peace on earth can be. Reconciliation of peoples to become a caring, sharing community demanded that they live in the spirit of the reconciliation of human diversities, and that, in turn, mandated continual, even daily, forgiveness of one another their faults. As St. Paul put it: "Bear one another's burdens, and in this way you will fulfill the law of Christ" (Galatians 6:2).

The priority the Bible gives to reconciliation among people, even over recovery from a physical disability or a mortal illness, is something physicians and those in the various pastoral ministries that deal with sicknesses of all sorts must keep in mind. They may encounter in patients a deeper malaise than the physical maladies that torment them. A vital connection exists between reconciliation and healing. The healing that ensues on moral forgiveness and inner reconciliation enables us to live out the restored relationships to the fullest. At times the cause of the illness may, indeed, be the stress that weakens one's immune system making the patient more susceptible to diseases otherwise kept at bay by the body's natural defenses. The physician may wonder what is eating away at the patient beneath the physical surface of the illness. When the medical practice is open to the kind of relationship in trust that can take place when doctors pray with and for their patients, the inner reconciliation that such a relationship promotes may, in turn, create a powerful stimulus to the body's defenses to rejoin the battle for health and life.

OUR JOURNEYS IN FAITH

Though we come from separate denominations, both Bill and I were born into a common Judeo-Christian religious tradition. We were nurtured in Sunday school (Bill), in parochial religious instruction (me). Both of us heard the stories of the heroic figures of the Bible and their power with the Lord God who created us all. We absorbed with interest the heroism of Samson, Samuel, King David, the prophets, and of course, the stories of Jesus. Though we both acknowledge Jesus as our Savior, Lord, and Brother, it would be accurate to say we had only hazy ideas of what those titles meant during our growing years. We learned how to define the terminology pertaining to God, Jesus, Spirit, Trinity, Incarnation, how to recite the creeds, and to believe that we knew and understood God. We were awarded with words of praise and acceptance into the cycles of church affiliation, such as communion and confirmation, if we could repeat these formulae accurately to the satisfaction of our dedicated teachers: the volunteer teachers of Bill's Sunday school sessions or, in my case, the saintly nuns of Most Blessed Sacrament Elementary School or MBS (which we had irreverently dubbed "Mary's Beauty Shop"). Perhaps the only doubt that entered my mind occurred when at the end of one school year I proudly brought home the Religion Medal for being the outstanding student in religion. My mother accepted it with a smile while adding: "You're lucky they didn't test you on obedience!" Bill claims the only prize he ever won in religion was for attendance!

Only later would we acquire some degree of theological sophistication, Bill at Princeton University and I at schools run by the De La Salle Christian Brothers, a religious order that I joined at the immature age of fifteen, too young to sow any wild oats, yet old enough to believe that I knew just about everything dealing with the Catholic faith. Knowledge of religion was my strength—so I thought. Somehow the simplicity of our earlier religious upbringing never seemed to leave us. This included supreme confidence in the power of prayer, whether it was for success in exams, the speedy recovery of a sick person, team success in the big game or swimming meet, or even the seemingly impossible. When Bill's father died at age forty-one, Bill's mother, a teacher, began reading to him a spiritual collection *(Daily Word)* which he has continued to read until this day. He learned that affirmative prayer helped him in his own life and later helped him in praying with and for his patients. Did we both ever pray for help, Bill in the course of Physics 101 preparing for medical school, and I in the New York Regents Exams so I could win advanced placement at La Salle College? Did we both pray for the restoration to health of a loved one whose medical history indicated a terminal illness? Yes to both of these questions.

Our faith was truly simplistic in its expression. Only when we both experienced the utter futility of our own efforts to control our lives, and to make events work to our advantage, did we really learn to pray. Yes, we knew that prayer was defined as the lifting up of our minds and hearts to God, that prayer was a conversation with our Father God who cares for us, with our brother Jesus who saved us, and with and actually through their Spirit of love who makes our prayer possible in the first place. But did our prayer life ever grow beyond the superficial? If marriages die the death of failure to communicate with each other, prayer certainly dies the death of self-centered "gimme this and gimme that." When Bill's first marriage unexpectedly ended, and when my daughter was at death's antechamber, so to speak, we both began to understand our own failures to enter into a genuine relationship with the God ever near, ever listening, ever more intimate to us than we are to ourselves, as St. Augustine once confessed in a moment of spiritual awakening.[8]

We had read the Bible, but we never fully understood those inspired words as more than boosts to our professed faith in our given churches. We believed in the veracity of the Bible and in the preachings and teachings of our churches; therefore, we were "in the truth." Pity those not so blessed! Yet, those stories, those words, so often proclaimed as sacred, inspired texts and Bible teachings, guaranteed with none other than divinely invested inerrancy, were swallowed like a communion wafer but never digested as God's special word for us. We learned something about God, but a whole lot more about ourselves and the way in which God becomes intimate in our personal lives through joys and, in a paradoxical way, through sadness and suffering. Luther said it well when he declared that God's word in itself was nothing, but when God's word became God's word *for me,* this was everything. In a way, a significant part of this book is a story of how God's word became God's word for both of us and how we both learned how to pray and what faith demanded of us.

FURTHER REFLECTIONS: DOCTOR BILL

In my own life I had what one might call with some exaggeration a "near-death" experience and a deliverance that I attribute not to luck but to an intervention by God. It was March 1946, and a typical bleak day on the North Atlantic with its accompanying rough sea. I was third officer in charge of the 12:00 to 4:00 watch (midnight to 4:00 a.m., noon to 4:00 p.m.) on a Navy troop transport. Our mission was to transport 1,500 German and Italian prisoners of war from their camps in the United States to Europe and then to bring 1,500 American troops back to the United States. This operation was repeated a number of times. But one specific event during this trip to Europe has remained etched in my memory. Although I had made only twelve Atlantic crossings at the time, I felt I knew a lot about the sea. I was only nineteen years old at the time, but I felt confident about carrying out my responsibilities. The ship was pitching, sending up sheets of spray that washed over the wheelhouse. When ships are underway, the custom is to keep the door facing the windward side of the wheelhouse closed, while the other door, on the leeward side, usually remained open. A railing inside the wheelhouse of every ship extends the width of this area in order to grasp if need be. It is located just below a series of windows facing the bow. The windows are used to track the ship's direction and locate any activity going on in the ship's vicinity, such as icebergs, other ships, buoys, land, lighthouses, even floating mines in those days. As I casually stood, resting my weight primarily on one leg, and loosely grasping the railing in the wheelhouse, the ship suddenly did a forty-degree roll, propelling me across the wheelhouse. I found myself heading for the open door. The rough sea, it only a few feet away, seemed eager to welcome me. Off-balance and virtually flying across the wheelhouse, I grabbed the metal doorframe surrounding the open door and held on until the ship rolled back the other way. I learned something that day: expect the unexpected in rough weather. One may say that was "lucky"—and in those days I probably did. But I now look at the sudden surge of strength to hold on for dear life, not as an adrenaline impulsion from my fear of dying, but as a strength coming from God's providential care watching over me. Knowing as only God can, of how one day I might be an instrument in God's providing care to many others through my medical ministry, God intervened on my behalf. Could I have been rescued had I let go? Some time later, I realized that lowering a lifeboat into those mountainous waves would have been hazardous and probably unsuccessful. Now, years later, when recalling the incident, I thank God for that act of deliverance and I can better appreciate the words of the Psalmist: "God is our refuge and strength, a very present help in trouble. Therefore we will not fear . . . in the heart of the sea, though its waters roar and foam" (Psalm 46:1-3).

On another occasion, I might have died had it not been for another divine intervention that kept me alive. The year was 1956. I was ending a month's leave in Europe and was standing in line at the Air Force base in Frankfort, Germany, hoping to hitch a free ride back to the States. Often there was "space available"—a few empty seats that could be occupied on a first come, first served, basis. About a dozen other servicemen were ahead of me. It was the end of a month's leave following a sizable number of Atlantic crossings as the ship's medical officer. I sensed a certain uneasiness, frequently looking at my wristwatch while at the same time watching the length of the line of waiting servicemen ahead of me. It soon became apparent that time was moving more quickly than the line ahead of me. I had to report back to New York. If time ran out, I would be AWOL (absent without official leave), not a pleasant thought for a serviceman. Decision time came when only a few men were ahead of me, but I couldn't wait any longer, so I paid $300 and boarded a commercial airliner.

The moment the plane landed in New York, I was astonished and saddened to see the headlines in the papers: MATS [Military Air Transport Service] PLANE DOWN OFF THE AZORES; ALL 69 ABOARD LOST. Upon reflection, I can say that the impulse not to wait any longer and to take a commercial flight back to the States was another instance when the Lord intervened, through my own anxiety, to keep me away from that doomed flight. I grieved for those who were lost, but I cannot help thinking that God moved me to take the commercial flight because of some design for my future that would affect someone else in need. I could only wonder what God had in mind for me at that mysterious later time.

I thought of that incident when I was of some help to a patient named Harry. Harry had been employed by a large pharmaceutical company as a research chemist, but sadly enough, he disliked his job. Having completed nineteen years with the same company, he struggled to finish out the last year, looking forward to a nice retirement package. But before reaching the retirement goal, he was "downsized" and let go. Harry was devastated. I remember praying with Harry soon after he lost his job, thanking God in advance for already starting a process that would allow him to fully use his gifts in some other situation. That initial "disaster" turned out to be the best thing that could have happened to him. After a short time, he started his own small company, and by the end of a few years, Harry had hired over a dozen employees. He was working seventy hours a week, instead of the previous forty, but loving every day of work.

I cannot help but think of how many have experienced similar losses that have become gains. The challenge in our spiritual relationship with God is to remain trustful that God will be present within us to help us through them. With ever-deepening faith in God's love and grace, even tough times can promote spiritual growth and an ever increasing consciousness of God's providential care of us.

Because of the mysteriousness of how God intervenes in our lives, how God leads us to do what God wants of us, despite the difficulties and puzzles of discerning just what that might be, I love to read the prophet Jeremiah and take his advice to heart. He likewise emphasizes that we must trust in the only true God who made the earth filled with wisdom, power, and justice rather than putting our trust in "false gods" (Jeremiah 10:10-12). From ancient times to the present, the world in general and people such as me have been exposed to many "false gods." I include our materialism, our excessive patriotism, and our insensitivity to the poor around us as among those "false gods." We cannot forget the way Adolph Hitler, the Nazi dictator, became like a "god" in Nazi Germany as an example of what can happen to us as a people. Nor can we forget how some Americans can set up for themselves the false gods of money, status, and domination over others. Throughout the psalms one finds the *true* God who is always present and trustworthy but who disturbs our peace with the challenges to promote peace, justice, and compassion.

Both Geff and I have shared hours of discussion in and out of class over the impact Jesus' faith has had on us and over how God has intervened in our lives. Jesus, too, has disturbed our peace with the incessant demands he places on us through the Sermon on the Mount and his vision of what counts at the final judgment on our lives. Jesus' making common cause with sinners, his courage in confronting evil in high places and among the political and religiously powerful, have given us challenges that disturb our residues of complacency. We especially drew inspiration from Jesus' compassion for the sick and the downtrodden in the light of the Gospels and because of our respective vocations as physician and theologian-teacher with responsibilities to our patients and students to be more Christlike.

PRAYER WITH PATIENTS: DOCTOR BILL

Despite the many stories I have told of how my praying with and for my patients has been so helpful to me in my own health care ministry, it was not easy for me to get to the point of praying with someone. It was initially a barrier that I crossed only with trepidation and hope. Reaching that point in my prayer life during my career as a healer came about gradually. I knew firsthand from my training as a physician that people everywhere are hurting. Regardless of their backgrounds, people are crying out to be listened to, to be cared for, to be healed. I knew in my heart and from my own experience of sadness and loneliness, when prayer seemed to be all that I had going for me, that patients want an ear that listens and a heart that understands and is attentive to their needs. I had come to the realization that health care providers must react with compassion and not just with empty sympathy. We have to lighten our patients' yokes. We have to be present to them with our hearts and not just our scientific minds. Chuck Swindoll, a noted Christian writer, touched on this when he wrote, "When people are hurting, they need much more than an accurate analysis and diagnosis."[9] Our spiritual natures must be able to communicate with their spiritual natures—we must attempt to feel a oneness with each patient.

At times, I have sensed that no words needed to be said; just being present with the patient could by itself be a prayer. But, whether through intuition or discernment, I have never had a patient say "No" when asked if we could pray together about a specific concern. I discovered that I had to go through three stages, each separated by weeks or longer, to reach the ultimate stage, of praying together *with* someone.[10] Before doing this, note that it is my conviction that our God wants us to be whole in our bonding one with another; second, I believe that God always hears our prayers.

The first stage of my journey using prayer as an adjunct to medical practice began with the hospital discharge of Charles, a fifty-year-old bus driver recovering from a deep thrombophlebitis in the calf of his leg. His hospital stay was happily over; he was now well enough to go home. Discerning that he was a prayerful person, I summoned enough courage to remark, "Charles, as you know, this is the moment you were looking forward to; you're going home today. But I wanted to let you know that I was praying for your complete recovery every day while you were here." I held my breath as he replied in a very straightforward fashion, "Thank you very much. I appreciate that." Whew! He did not criticize me for stepping over the familiar boundary of medical science into what I sensed to be the untested waters of things spiritual! Although I realized that caregivers are more effective by treating the "whole person" (mind, body, and spirit), it was a stretch to actually put this into action. It was an early attempt for me to meld science and faith into the healing process in a very real way. After many weeks had passed, I felt that I was ready to attempt the second stage of this "praying-with-patients journey."

Ellen illustrated the second stage for me. Unlike Charles, Ellen, a seventy-two-year-old widow, still required intravenous antibiotics for a severe pneumonia and was not yet ready for hospital discharge. With a number of intuitive insights and discernment received in the course of her hospital stay, I felt she was open to prayer. During a routine hospital visit, I was able to drum up enough courage to re-mark, "I hope you don't mind, but I've been praying for the healing of your pneumonia every night. I'm finding that prayer and science have a role to play in medical practice." Much to my great relief she re-plied, "Thank you very much. You see, I also believe in the power of prayer!" Under my breath I released a sigh of relief. I was elated at her response. My fear at this time was that a patient would castigate me for going into things spiritual, in areas beyond the boundaries of scientific medicine. I felt that a second step on the ladder had been accomplished.

Not too many weeks later, the time appeared ripe to climb the last step of this journey: praying *with* a patient. The catalyst for this last step was Henry, a forty-one-year-old man, a trained machinist, who was suffering from a heart attack. Upon completing the initial history, physical exam, and diagnostic tests, he suddenly turned to me and said, "Can I pray for you? You seem to be carrying a burden on your heart." My first reaction was shock! The roles had suddenly been turned. Logically I should have been praying for Henry; he was the one who was having a heart attack! Yet he was offering prayers for me! I admitted that I personally saw the power of prayer work in my personal life; I had sought God's help while undergoing a need for in-ner healing and certainly would appreciate a prayer. Upon hearing this, Henry immediately started to pray for my inner peace and con-tinued healing. Every day until discharge, Henry prayed for me. This, in turn, gave me the courage to pray at the same time for his recovery. We both realized that this was a new adventure for me as I struggled in prayer for the "right words" as I sat at his bedside.

It goes without saying, Henry was being closely monitored by my-self and all the CCU (cardiac care unit) staff during this time. Henry enjoyed a complete recovery and was soon discharged. Subsequently, we prayed for each other at every office visit. We had become "prayer partners" as well as continuing our professional doctor-patient relationship. Over time our prayers encompassed both medical and nonmedical issues. After several years, he received a very good job opportunity that required his moving to another state. It was apparent that we had served as channels for God's healing for each other.

Because of this experience, Henry served as a role model for me, and it was not too long before George, a sixty-eight-year-old retired civil engineer, was admitted for evaluation concerning a series of transient ischemic attacks (fleeting signs of an impending stroke). He was one of the first patients that inwardly encouraged me to leap to the third and last stage of my prayer journey. George made reference to the Lord, wore a cross around his neck, and sent out hints in routine conversation that he was a spiritual person. I asked if he would mind praying together, and call for God's healing presence in addition to all that science could offer. As with so many of us who are admitted for a potentially lethal illness, George was more than willing to actively bring God as a partner in the healing process. We then prayed together at the bedside, thanking God in advance for starting the healing process.

The third and final step had been reached! Since those early days, dozens of patients have become prayer partners with me, and they have added immeasurably to my own spiritual journey. What joy it has been and what wonderful relationships have been formed by *praying together.* Locations for prayer with patients (and friends) are limitless. Some examples that have worked include at the bedside, in the office, at home, in the hospital parking lot, or on the phone.

In some cases, however, I have felt the individual was *not* open for audible prayer. The stethoscope resting on the patient's chest is still a powerful channel for silent prayer when examining him or her. Discernment is important. I have always tried to avoid spiritually "steamrolling" an unwilling patient or to appear to be proselytizing. Our religious beliefs are sacred and deserve respect. Sometimes, when dealing with varied cultural and ethnic backgrounds among medical students or among caregivers who may feel uncomfortable with audible prayer, I use another approach. I tell the patient, "I'll be thinking of you this morning during the surgery, and I will return later this afternoon to see how you are doing." This can be tantamount to a prayer.

Both Geff and I have read many books on spiritual healing. Geff has been reaffiliated with the De La Salle Christian Brothers through the Lasallian Leadership Institute of which he was the founding director. I became professed in the Third Order of St. Francis. I have been invited to give talks on inner healing in my medical practice to various secular and religious organizations. These now number well over a hundred invitations, in all of which I feel that God is somehow working through me. New doors were opening with patients, family, and friends. My life was being turned around in a profoundly different way. The bricks that I had built up to protect the vulnerability of this well-trained scientist have been fast disappearing and the joy of my opening myself up to the inner hurts of others brought home more powerfully than ever before the importance of treating the whole person in the practice of medicine.[11]

Being honest and vulnerable ourselves in the many talks that Geff and I give about healing and prayer from our perspectives as a physician and theologian creates a certain credibility. The wonder of courage, humility, and the power of prayer becomes apparent to me when several in the audience come forward to share their faith through the many ways in which God has answered prayers for them. Sometimes, too, these people of faith require and request further prayers for themselves, their family, or their friends. I am convinced that the openness of those in these groups is a response to the openness of the caregivers' sharing of God's own work within them.

We end this chapter with a pause rather than a conclusion. In the next chapters we will explore the nature and power of faith and prayer and their importance in extending our compassion to the sick and needy in the health care ministry.

DISCUSSION QUESTIONS

1. Does the fact that physicians pray for and, in some cases, pray with their patients, detract from or enhance their medical practice? Explain.
2. Dr. Haynes states that praying *with* someone can sometimes have a healing quality greater than praying *for* someone. Do you agree?
3. How does the story of Helen illustrate the healing power of prayer in the practice of medicine?
4. Do the divine gifts of faith, hope, and love help us become more loving and compassionate in our dealings with others? How do individuals experience the gifts of faith, hope, and love?
5. An awakening and renewal of faith or a yearning for a deeper meaning of life beyond the signs or totems of our material success is happening. Can you identify the signs?
6. Is God involved in all healing whether physical, emotional, or spiritual? Explain.

7. Discuss the difference between a healing and a cure, as claimed by the authors.
8. In what sense can a spiritual healing be more important than a physical cure?
9. Comment on the authors' journeys in faith and describe your own journey to a more mature, adult faith?
10. Comment on the three stages Dr. Haynes explains in his becoming a prayer partner with his patients. Can this be applied to other aspects of health care?

Chapter 2

Faith: Its Nature and Its Work Among the Sick and Needy

Randolph Byrd, a San Francisco cardiologist, found that patients admitted to the Critical Care Unit in a San Francisco hospital, who were prayed for by individuals several miles away, did better than those control patients where the subject of prayer was not mentioned. Of course, the patients who were prayed for gave their permission for this prayerful intervention; and what is important, they were aware that prayers for their recovery were being offered daily. It is our contention in these pages that prayers can favorably affect the whole person—the individual's mind, body, and spirit, and in biochemical ways as well. More will be said about this; but we have become convinced that, when we know someone is praying for us daily, even on the opposite coast of the country, we can experience an inner peace, a warm feeling that we have interpreted as the power of the Spirit at work within us.

The results of Byrd's study reveal that the group for whom prayers were offered had a shorter hospital stay, had fewer problems with rhythm disorders, less heart failure, less need for antibiotics, fewer episodes of pneumonia, and were less frequently intubated and ventilated. This study suggests that intercessory prayer to our God does have a favorable effect on a patient's medical condition.[1]

A 1996 study done in Israel likewise confirms our conviction about the power of prayer in maintaining good bodily health. Scientists there compared 3,900 people living in Kibbutzim more than sixteen years and found a 40 percent decrease in deaths from cardiovascular disease among the religious when compared to a control group of secular peers.[2] A Maryland study of 92,000 residents found that regular churchgoers (at least once a week) had significantly fewer deaths

Is There a God in Health Care?
© 2006 by The Haworth Press, Inc. All rights reserved.
doi:10.1300/5554_02

from heart disease, emphysema, cirrhosis, and suicide.[3] An increasing amount of data suggest those with deep religious convictions and a strong faith fare better medically than their nonreligious, nonbelieving peers. A host of other published studies have similar outcomes.

These findings suggest that inner peace relates in a biochemical way to the immune system and healing as well. The T cells in the blood are elevated and are related to an increased immune system and better healing when an individual enjoys inner peace. On the other hand, other blood elements (e.g., interleukin-1 and -6) may cause inflammation, and decrease the body's immune system, thereby delaying healing. These harmful agents will be found in the bloodstream when an individual is lacking inner peace and remains in an agitated state. This should be exciting information for all caregivers. Physicians who may feel uncomfortable praying for their patients may then be encouraged to either tell the patients that they will be thinking of them or they could call the local pastor or rabbi or hospital chaplain knowing that their patient's condition may very well benefit from prayer. This is not to suggest that the power of prayer inspirited by faith now becomes merely one more weapon in the *medical* arsenal alone. We are advocating, rather, the integration into one's daily life of the faith that is God's gift for the taking. This is the holistic power of God's Spirit which promotes both physical and spiritual healing. At times, this power extends to a different kind of healing, that of a resignation and acceptance of death. This faith is conducive to the peace of mind that is also God's gift at the climactic moment of life, a terminally ill person's entrance into beatific destiny.

THE NATURE AND ROLE OF FAITH
IN A LIFE WORTH LIVING

The benefits of everyday living of one's faith are, indeed, enormous in terms of emotional and physical health, but the very idea that we need to have faith to experience healing of our ills opens us up to the larger question: What is this faith? We might be prompted to ask the allied question of whether we have the kind of faith that is praised in the Bible. This is the same faith that one finds exemplified in the lives of the saints and is preached in religious services as that divine gift that justifies us, puts us on the road to sanctification, and heals us in sickness. Some modern-day healers—often called "miracle workers" even over their objections—are diffident about the faith healings shown on TV that are impressive for their sheer drama.

The famed priest healer Father Ralph DiOrio, for example, expresses his disdain for such healings, arguing that they can easily be confused with genuine divine healing because they place too much emphasis on the strength of faith of the sufferer. To him there seems to be too much human calculation, suggestiveness, and emotional oratory in the process. He believes that healings depicted on TV are more the result of psychosomatic influence and rousing histrionics than the divine healing based on God's providential care. "What we need to preach in divine healing," he writes, "is the message of God's love, the episodes of Gospel stories, the compassion of Jesus toward sinners and toward the sick, the offering of God's love as our hope for redemption."[4]

Faith is never easy to define, and often enough faith is confused with religious practice and even moral self-righteousness. One of the most intriguing aspects of the Gospels, as they narrate the miracles of Jesus, is their insistence on faith as the power effecting the cures that people have requested of Jesus. Jesus, in turn, is often quoted as attributing to the faith of the petitioner the healing power that passes through him. "Your faith has made you well" (Matthew 9:22), Jesus declared to the woman who touched the hem of his garment in hopes of a cure. In another passage Jesus tells the blind man by the roadside, "Receive your sight; your faith has healed you" (Luke 18:42). In Jesus' driving an evil spirit from the body of a young boy, the lad's father begs Jesus to cure his son of this spiritual affliction only to be told that "everything is possible to the one who believes." The father's answer is captivating because so many readers of the Bible resonate with it: "I believe; help my unbelief!" (Mark 9:24). And, in the letter of James, Christians are told that "the prayer of faith will save the sick" (James 5:15).

If these scriptural passages are clear on the need for faith in the healing process, the impression is strengthened by what one sees on television when the TV healers are shown preaching faith, asking for testimonies of what faith has done for individuals, and demanding of those who come forth that they have the faith which alone can work the cure—of course, with considerable input from the preacher who has led the sick people to profess their faith in the powers of God's Spirit to overcome any illness. Those wonders in the full view of

thousands give homage to the power of God to affect a dramatic healing in just about any place and at any time, even the gaze of the many
who watch the show with interest. But the very drama of the public
passage from sickness to health through the power of a faith healing
brings up once again the question of just what kind of faith is so
effective.

The healings depicted in the Gospels and throughout history do indeed speak of faith as God's gift that brings healing and salvation.
This explains in part why people continue to ponder the nature of this
great gift, especially in times when they have been told that, if they
have faith, all things are possible, including the healing they desire.
Later we speak of instances when it is equally clear that no apparent
faith was present prior to the seeming miraculous cure of an illness.
Does God's power in the divine interventions to heal the sick depend
on the person's disposition of faith? Can God send Spirit into the soul
of a nonbeliever with the same results as documented in so-called
faith-based healings? Or, to borrow a speculation by Francis Mac-
Nutt, does God heal the nonbeliever as the preliminary step in the
eventual advent of genuine religious faith in that person?[5] Obviously,
we are again confronted with the mystery of God's miraculous power
bestowed not when we will but at the unpredictable decisions of the
God who, as Augustine has claimed, is intimate to us and knows us
better than we know ourselves.[6] Often the faith we attempt to describe in this chapter is conjoined to prayer in the reciprocal way in
which faith moves us to pray, and prayer, in turn, nurtures the faith
that infuses human life with transcendental meaning.

It is easy simply to give an all-embracing definition of faith that is
theologically sound and categorically approved by the mainstream
religions. However, we are convinced that cold definitions do little to
help us appreciate the manner in which God's gift of faith takes on
such manifold experiential expressions in the individuals whose lives
tell us more about the nature of faith through its effects than any textbook definition. What follows is a selection of theological reflections
on faith backed up by stories of people who have exemplified a life of
faith that has made an impact on contemporary society with all its ills.
This includes the victimization of so many vulnerable people who cry
to God for their deliverance.

FAITH AS A PERSON TO WHOM WE COMMIT OURSELVES IRREVOCABLY

As with St. Paul before him who wrote, "For to me, living is Christ and dying is gain" (Philippians 1:21), Søren Kierkegaard saw Christian faith not as a doctrine but as a person to whom we commit ourselves irrevocably.[7] Kierkegaard also argues that faith as commitment to God is, at face value, an absurdity since it brings God who is totally other into a communion of love with a creature who is sinful. This is a relationship not of equals, but of a powerful deity deliberately becoming vulnerable in drawing close to one who is a sinner but now elevated into likeness with a caring Lord. The paradox is such that the elements of absurdity fade away through the interiority of personal faith. But this faith, which overcomes the puzzle of a mighty God creating intimacy through trust with an unworthy human sinner, is nonetheless for believers a leap into the unknown where the only certainty is trust in the beloved. In this way Kierkegaard likens faith to the trust that only a genuine love can generate. Hence for him the "leap of faith is the risk of love."[8] Kierkegaard is not uncomfortable with the intrusion of doubts in one's faith, but he is suspicious of attempts to portray faith as a dogma, or law, or a rationalized apologetic. Faith is ultimately the trust that can exist only between lovers who can take the risk of entrusting themselves totally to each other. Jesus' prayer telling his Father God that not his but the Father's will be done is an expression of such faith.

TILLICH AND FAITH AS ONE'S ULTIMATE CONCERN

If Kierkegaard sees faith as a leap that stretches the potential for love and trust within people, theologian Paul Tillich claims that everyone has a faith of sorts since faith is an essential dynamic of human existence. Faith for him is nothing other than one's "ultimate concern," and one's faith is defined by the concerns into which one invests ultimacy. Tillich understands faith as a centered act of the whole personality that demands one's total surrender and promises total fulfillment. In terms of this "ultimate concern," he goes on, people are driven to reject every other claim on their energies. He sees faith as a generic of the human condition that is specified by the choices we make and the various directions our lives assume. Tillich's analysis makes it clear why so many people claim allegiance to a particular religious denomination while their behavior may be contradictory of the values they publicly profess to accept. In the Hitler era, for example, many churchgoers were such avid nationalists that their allegiance seemed more directed to Adolf Hitler than to Jesus Christ.

For Tillich, who had fled Nazism in his native Germany, their real faith was nationalism or even the histrionic patriotism that Hitler inspired in the masses. In the present age many Americans profess to be followers of Jesus Christ, yet they are unflagging in support of wars and the death penalty and neglectful of the poor, all actions and attitudes that contradict the teachings of Jesus. Many self-proclaimed Christians are so supportive of war that they vilify the pacifists whose stance is close to the nonviolence that Jesus exemplified. Likewise there are those whose "ultimate concern" is pursuing the icons of money, economic success, and social standing. Tillich is adamant that these aspects of our competitive Western culture are in essence the dimensions of their real faith, not Jesus Christ whom they might laud in their creeds and liturgies. Only when people can see all the false gods that creep into their sense of meaning and fulfillment as ultimately very limited, transitory, and unfulfilling might they be open to the true ultimate and converted from their "idolatrous faith."

If Tillich is correct, it is easy to understand why an idolatrous faith is hardly aligned with the loving trust of a purified religious faith. Tillich's analysis of faith, seen against the backdrop of the German and American nationalism he opposed and the crass materialism and secularism of America that he criticized as idolatrous, is sobering to those whose concerns are less than ultimate. His thoughts are important when one is faced with an illness that is terminal. Prayer, in that context, is a reminder that God is the ultimate end of every act of faith and of every path leading to life eternal, even when that path meanders into byroads of suffering and death.

Tillich notes that the ultimate consequence of a life in pursuit of the idols that masquerade as genuine faith is existential disappointment and demonic despair. The way out is, of course, the awakening that unfortunately often springs from the heartache of having worshipped false gods and being frustrated at their inability to satisfy one's longing for human fulfillment. For some, the experience of illness or even death may provide the moment of awakening. Such a conversion, even if it is a deathbed moment of awareness, is itself a healing. What are called "deathbed conversions" may, indeed, have the power to open one's eyes to episodes in life that have been squandered in the hunt for dehumanizing goals. A deathbed conversion could set the sufferer on a new path to a faith where the truth of the Lord can be found, even if only for the brief time one has left to live. The healings that line the pages of the Gospels are themselves stories of new pathways to the peace of mind that Jesus opened for his followers in his statements about those who are truly blessed (Matthew 5:1-16).[9]

FAITH AS THAT FOR WHICH WE WOULD RISK OUR LIVES

What Tillich has called idolatrous faith, Dietrich Bonhoeffer depicts as the consequence of pursuing "cheap grace." This cheapening of faith yields an easy Christianity in which one takes comfort in having been baptized and certified as a churchgoer, despite not ever having lived according to the teachings of Jesus Christ. This is the superficial faith that Bonhoeffer claims exists when so-called Christians receive absolution for sins but never have to do any real penance or seek God's forgiveness. In that kind of faith individuals can have the social status of being true believers but can pick and choose which demands of Christ they will respect and which ones they will set aside because they interfere with concerns or ideologies that are not supported by gospel values. The attitudes that Bonhoeffer excoriates are those that prefer the bargain-basement way of being Christian rather than the challenges of Jesus Christ. Jesus urged his followers to walk in the ways of social justice, contribute to peace on earth, and exercise compassion toward the handicapped. Bonhoeffer's lament that Germans made Adolf Hitler their conscience and not Jesus Christ[10] has been repeated whenever Christians follow the dictates of political leaders who capitalize on neglecting the most vulnerable of their citizens and pandering to the idols of racial hatred, militarism, and blind patriotism. Such was the Hitler legacy that had mesmerized so many ordinary German citizens. Such are the dangers to genuine faith whenever the Gospel is cheapened and faith turned into an idolatry.

Before his execution, Bonhoeffer described faith as the willing-ness to risk one's life for the values that Jesus Christ taught. In a letter to his fellow conspirators in their plot to assassinate Adolf Hitler and bring an end to the killing fields of World War II, he reminded them that faith demands they not be merely bystanders as evil was being done by the Nazi government. Their faith, he told them, meant that they needed to

> have some share in Christ's large-heartedness by acting with re-sponsibility and in freedom when the hour of danger comes, and by showing a real compassion that springs, not from fear, but from the liberating and redeeming love of Christ for all who suf-fer. Mere waiting and looking on is not Christian behavior.[11]

The day after the failure of the assassination attempt and less than a year before his execution on April 9, 1945, he recounted for his best friend, Eberhard Bethge, a conversation he had had with the French pacifist Jean Lasserre. They had chatted about what they wanted to do with their lives. Lasserre said he would like to become a saint. Bon-hoeffer replied that he would like to learn to have faith. He thought then that this would mean he had "to live a holy life, or something like it." However, in prison, he had found his answer:

> I'm still discovering right up to this moment, that it is only by living completely in this world that one learns to have faith. . . . By this worldliness I mean living unreservedly in life's duties, problems, successes and failures, experiences and perplexities. In so doing we throw ourselves completely into the arms of God, taking seriously, not our own sufferings, but those of God in the world. . . . That, I think, is faith; . . . and that is how one be-comes a human being and a Christian (cf. Jer. 45!). How can success make us arrogant, or failure lead us astray, when we share in God's sufferings through a life of this kind?[12]

Bonhoeffer's letter, though written in an entirely different context, could very well be a statement of the faith demanded of those in the healing professions. They too must live "unreservedly in life's duties, problems, successes and failures, experiences and perplexities."

In one of his final letters before being transferred to the more tightly controlled Gestapo prison, Bonhoeffer declared that faith for him was nothing less than participation in the being of Jesus, the man for others. He added that in faith we often ask the wrong questions, such as what must we believe or what can we believe, rather than the test case of just how genuine our faith really is: "What do we really believe? I mean, believe in such a way that we stake our lives on it?"[13] The continuing fascination with the life and writings of Bonhoeffer can be traced to his not merely teaching about faith but to the fact that he lived out his convictions, risking his freedom and life to bring an end to the evils of Nazism that had created the death camps and brought the world into the bloodiest conflict of the twentieth century.

One way of looking at faith is that it is not merely a gift of God openly bestowed at religious rites of initiation, but also as a divinely given power from within that needs to be cultivated. Faith is meant to be our way of living—we are to live by faith and not by the empirical evidence that our scientific age seeks as validation of beliefs. So as we accept the gift of faith, we are then asked to apply it in our lifetime by surrendering ourselves to what God would have us be and do. How extensive could those demands become? If Dietrich Bonhoeffer's classic study of Christian discipleship is any gauge, following Christ in the way of the Gospel could lead to death at the hands of the forces of oppression. "Whenever Christ calls us, his call leads us to death," he wrote.[14] At times, faith in Christ could become the demand that we repudiate what our contemporary society would exalt as our idealized self, often measured by our material accumulations or our monetary achievements. For some, possessed by their possessions, worshipping the icon of self-exaltation, that could become a kind of living death. In faith we make ourselves available to do what God wants as discerned in the scriptural and meditative sources of our religious affiliation. We have a wonderful heritage of faith that helps us to discern those "plans." And, once discovered and once accepted, we are enabled to pass this on to our descendants as a legacy of a humanizing and divinizing tradition that proclaims God's goodness and providential care.

FAITH AS A LONGING FOR GOD

The presence in our lives of a caring God has its counterpart in our longing to be with and follow the paths to love such a God in return.

This longing inspired the great theologian Karl Rahner to describe faith as much more than orthodoxic correctness or theological formulae petrified for all times despite the changing nature of language, culture and history. Faith for Rahner was considered one's gifted orientation to the holy, incomprehensible mystery of God. Rahner likened faith to a sword that pierces our soul.

> Faith is the enduring of this sword, and so the refusal to think precipitously of being reconciled, the readiness to live on hope in the depths with the conflict which reaches down into the fragmentariness and unintegratability of our existence, to the point . . . at which the human being can only do one thing: to despair or to entrust itself unconditionally to that mysterious unity and reconciliation we call God. Faith is many things: peace, liberty, trust, joy, and much more.[15]

Rahner insists that God has implanted a detectable hunger in us, moving us to believe in something, to make sense of our lives. Similar to Rahner's concerns, the noted psychologist Eugene Kennedy contends that as we respond to life's many responsibilities, the door of faith opens further, allowing us to focus better on the meaning of our life and its significance in the world—this helps us to understand the reason we are here, to derive the purpose of our human experience here on earth, and how it fits with the designs of God on each of us.[16]

FAITH THAT SUSTAINS IN THE MIDST OF SUFFERING: ERNEST GORDON

Faith can provide the perseverance as well as the spiritual and emotional sustenance to survive extreme anguish and pain. This faith can be illustrated by a friend who survived intense suffering in a Japanese prison camp. Ernest Gordon, former dean of the Princeton University Chapel, served in Sumatra as a commander of a Scottish Highlander regiment in February 1943. He was on the verge of being cut off by a large contingent of Japanese soldiers when he and nine other men escaped in a small boat. Traveling at night, they attempted to get to the Allied lines, but before reaching their goal, and after spending two months at sea, they were captured by a Japanese patrol boat.

Ernest spent the next three and a half years in various Japanese prison camps. In his book, *Through the Valley of the Kwai,* he describes his experiences as a prisoner involved in the building of the railroad bridge over the River Kwai. "The Japanese," he wrote,

> had special refinements for those prisoners who did not comply with certain orders. Some were tortured by having their heads crushed in vises; some were filled up with water and then jumped upon; some were tied to a tree by their thumbs; some were buried alive in the ground. . . .[17]

Eventually conditions became so bad that the rule of the jungle, "look out for oneself," seemed the only way to survive. Then cholera struck the camps, and many more died from lack of medical attention. Religion as a crutch was tried during the early months, but, because it seemed too much like an unreal prop, it failed, nor did the prayers they offered bring any relief from their frustrations. They felt that they were forsaken prisoners with no hope. Gordon suffered from dysentery and beriberi; eventually his legs were no longer able to support him.

As they were moved from one camp to another, it became apparent that selfishness, greed, and hatred were seen as antilife, while love, self-sacrifice, and mercy were seen as the only real expressions of faith and support now given by God to the prisoners. Bible study groups were held, prisoners began helping those who were worse off, even giving up some of the meager food allotments. Two men took turns massaging Gordon's legs, devoting their spare energies in helping him to stand and then start to walk again. He recalled what developed in that prisoner camp.

> I was beginning to see that life was infinitely more complex, and at the same time more wonderful than I had ever imagined. True there was hatred, but there was also love. There was death, but there was also life. God had not left us. He was with us, calling us to live the divine life in fellowship.[18]

They were permitted to have discussion groups after work, and Gordon was chosen as the leader. "Through our readings and discussions we came to know Jesus. He was one of us." Jesus had undergone suffering also. They were slowly transformed from a mass of frightened people into a community.[19]

When liberated at the end of the war, Gordon had lost eighty pounds, and his waist measured eighteen inches. Reflecting on his years of captivity, however, he remarked:

> I knew the depths to which men could sink and the heights to which they could rise. I could speak knowledgeably of despair, but also of hope; of hatred, but also of love; of man without God, but of man sustained by God. I knew the power of the demonic, and I knew the greater power of the Holy Spirit.[20]

Faith ultimately sustained the survivors. God had showered the prisoners not with stylized prayers but with the strength of God's word and the acts of compassion one prisoner could show to another in worse straits. Love had conquered evil; life with God had even conquered death.

After the war Ernest went to a seminary in Edinburgh. Eventually he was called to be the dean of the Chapel at Princeton University. After serving for a number of years, he retired and immediately became very involved in an organization dedicated to restoring religious freedom in Russia. In 1990 he was elated to see that freedom of religion was finally made law in Russia. Many of the other communist countries soon followed suit.

In 1997 Gordon returned to Japan to visit the former Japanese officer responsible for many of the atrocities that the prisoners had accused him of permitting. Ernest's trip was a journey of faith; its purpose was to offer forgiveness to the Japanese commandant and to attempt a reconciliation. The meeting was successful; a heart filled with bitterness of many decades was replaced with an inner peace and the warmth of the reconciliation of two erstwhile enemies. The issue has now been closed. Faith had sustained Gordon throughout his horrible prison experiences. The Spirit then led him to the ministry and eventually to ordination. Upon retirement his faith kept moving him to preach God's word, to comfort those hurting, and to be an inspiration to those who were his pastoral ministry. He died peacefully in Princeton in January 2002.

FAITH AS "LETTING GO" OF EVERYTHING STANDING BETWEEN US AND GOD: CARDINAL BERNARDIN

Gordon's story was a fascinating journey from intense suffering and near despair to the peace that came from the faith, prayers, and acts of compassion that brought hope into the bleak conditions of his imprisonment. A different journey in faith was that lived by Joseph Cardinal Bernardin, the widely admired Archbishop of Chicago, who died in 1997. Terminally ill and reflecting on his past life as a spiritual journey back to God, Bernardin described the turning point in his faith as a "letting go." It took him many years, he confesses, to cease grasping all those things, material possessions and administrative trivia, that had kept him from an intimate relationship with Jesus Christ. Despite his long years in seminary formation and more than twenty years as a busy priest, he finally realized that his life's priority consisted of doing good deeds yet never setting aside the adequate time needed for personal prayer. It was only when he asked three young priests for help in praying that he received from the Lord through them the challenge to practice what he had been preaching and to give quality time to God in prayer by putting aside the first hour of the day for God, no matter what. Through a small book, he shared with his people the unbelievable "gift of peace" he received in return for this surrender of his time to the Lord. He does not gloss over the difficulties encountered when remaining faithful to this discipline in the practice and nourishment of his faith.

> Still, letting go is never easy. I have prayed and struggled constantly to be able to let go of things more willing, to be free of everything that keeps the Lord from finding greater hospitality in my soul or interferes with my surrender to what God asks of me. It is clear that God wants me to let go now. But there is something in us humans that makes us want to hold onto ourselves and everything and everybody familiar to us. . . . So I now let go more freely, delivered by the Lord from the frustration I sometimes experienced even when I tried before, as earnestly as I could, to break free from the grip of things.[21]

Faith as a "letting go" of everything standing between us and the giver of life and faith was for Bernardin the source of the strength that amazed his friends. He was able to not only forgive a young man who had publicly slandered him, but also to welcome impending death from cancer as a friend. He was able to bring hope and joy into the lives of those who, like him, were in a life-and-death struggle against the lethal ravages of cancer. His story of how he came to welcome death as a friend has reached millions of readers offering them hope in what on the surface had appeared to be a hopeless situation. Death for him, as he claimed, would be the beginning of the eternal life to which he always aspired. The outpouring of gratitude for this ecclesiastic's inspiration has been captured on the film of his life that now serves as an inspiring story of personal faith and courage.[22]

FAITH AS THE INSPIRATION TO CARE
FOR THE NEEDY OF THIS WORLD: JEAN VANIER

An equally moving account of a journey in faith is that of Jean Vanier, founder of L'Arche, a worldwide network of communities whose mission is to care for mentally handicapped adults. One of the truly holy persons of our time, Vanier tells of his own relentless search for a sense of meaning in his life. Born into the prominent family of the nineteenth Governor General of Canada, he grew up in affluence. He became an officer in the Royal Canadian Navy while still in his twenties. Having resigned his commission in 1950, he undertook studies in philosophy and theology with a view toward ordination to the priesthood. He later dropped that plan and went on to complete work for a doctorate in philosophy from the Institut Catholique of Paris. His doctorate prepared him for a teaching career that lasted only a year. His search for Jesus continued, taking him to the village of Trosly where he was introduced to two mentally retarded men by Father Thomas Philippe, a compassionate Dominican priest whose life had been devoted to the handicapped. Father Philippe encouraged Vanier to become involved in the care of the two men, Raphael and Philippe. Vanier was deeply moved by the faith of this priest and inspired by the compassion he felt for the pain and abandonment Raphael and Philippe had suffered. Here was an outlet for his energies and here was where he could, perhaps for the first time in his life, encounter the Christ whom he had always wanted to follow. Vanier then purchased an old, dilapidated house in the village and took in these men, the first residents in the community of L'Arche, named after the image of the Ark that had provided refuge for the people of Noah's time and now a refuge for the mentally retarded. L'Arche was thus born in August 1964. Those who had suffered rejection at the hands of today's competitive society, where dignity was pegged to physical and financial achievements, were now accepted with full dignity into a community that cared.

Vanier does not romanticize the ministry of this community. In following Christ down this path of faith he had chosen to live with the handicapped whose spirit had often been broken as their dignity had been denied. For Vanier, this was where his journey in faith had led him and in L'Arche he had finally found Jesus Christ and meaning in his life. Caring for the mentally handicapped has its own challenge, as health caregivers of any age will attest. L'Arche was no exception. The mentally handicapped put Vanier and the caregivers of L'Arche in touch with their own inner pain where they could discover the broken parts of their own being. Vanier writes that this did not shake his faith. "I think the experiences of suffering enhanced my faith. Whatever caused me to touch my own inner pain made me realize I needed Jesus even more."[23]

Vanier is insistent that being a caregiver for these special people, despite their incessant demands on one's patience and energies, has the power to enhance our faith and strengthen our capacity to give love to others:

> The amazing thing about handicapped people is that they live on faith. Not just a religious faith, but faith in the sense of trust. Many of them have not developed their capacities of reason; so they live in a situation of trust. This is the foundation stone of the gift of faith. Religious faith comes easily to someone who lives on trust. And handicapped people live on faith. For somebody who lives on reason, though, faith is not very interesting or easy.[24]

Vanier notes, too, the simplicity and purity of the mentally handicapped, who live so close to the Beatitudes to which Jesus called his followers.

The documentary that captures the essence of Vanier's spirituality and the testimonies of those who have dedicated themselves to the ministry of caregiving with mentally handicapped adults provides a strong testimony to the claim that the mentally handicapped confer many unexpected blessings on them. In those relationships, so essential to maintaining the sense of personal dignity of every member of the L'Arche communities, the caregivers "experience a remarkable touch of love. And through that touch of love [they] feel a responsibility." He goes on to say that such

> love is an extraordinary reality; it is continually calling us forth. When we love others, we can walk with them and share their pain. I don't think that love means that we go to people just to cure them or to heal them—that can be a danger. We can be acting out of love for our own power. But as we enter into a relationship because we love the other person and we've been touched by that person, then we can share their pain.[25]

Faith for Vanier is the dynamic inspiriting of compassion for the handicapped. His words, though focused on his special ministry to the mentally handicapped, offer also a powerful statement of how this kind of spiritual outlook is related to the health care ministry. He insists that faith is easy when it goes along with a Jesus locked up in tabernacles of orthodoxic dogma, minimum observances and unbending rituals. At L'Arche they encounter a living Jesus. He calls the mentally handicapped the "barometer people" whose needs and the way we respond to people in need are the gauge of the true depths of our faith. His words are reminiscent of Bonhoeffer's claim that the only measure of our faith is that on which we stake our lives.[26]

FAITH AS THE INSPIRATION TO CARE FOR SOCIETY'S THROWAWAYS: MOTHER TERESA

Certainly one of the most widely known of saintly health caregivers is Mother Teresa of Calcutta. Similar to Jean Vanier, Mother Teresa's story has inspired many followers who are willing to embrace a life of evangelical poverty in order to tend to the sick and dying among the poor in far-flung regions of the world. She described her own journey in faith as a "call within a call" to found the Missionaries of Charity who would take a fourth vow, to offer free service in Christ's name to the poorest of the poor wherever they may be found.

And when that happens the only thing to do is to say "Yes." The message was quite clear—I was to give up all and follow Jesus into the slums—to serve him in the poorest of the poor. I knew it was his will and that I had to follow him.[27]

She had the extraordinary faith to look into the faces of dying, diseased beggars in the back streets of Calcutta and see the face of Jesus Christ in those who ached only for the one moment of love the sisters could give before death could release them from their misery. Mother Teresa picked up and cared for 40,000 abandoned people from the streets of Calcutta between 1952 and 1983. At the time of her death in 1997, at age eighty-seven, there were 168 houses of her religious order in India and hundreds more scattered among 105 countries.

To her sisters and to the world that would listen, she gave the following extraordinary testimony to her personal faith and the inspiration behind her mission.

Actually we are touching Christ's body in the poor. In the poor it is the hungry Christ that we are feeding, it is the naked Christ that we are clothing, it is to the homeless Christ that we are giving shelter. It is not just hunger for bread or the need of the naked for clothes or of the homeless for a house made of bricks. Even the rich are hungry for love, being cared for, for being wanted, for having someone to call their own.[28]

This statement of Mother Teresa could serve as a steady reminder of the nature of their vocation for health caregivers the world over. Many of these are themselves with the poor, outcasts, and handicapped in their respective communities.

The story of Mother Teresa captures what is arguably the major effect of faith in one's life, that of providing a vision in one's search for meaning in life that transcends the mundane and self-serving aspirations to which the average person is prone. Her example provoked considerable soul scrutiny on the part of the Church in presenting the Gospel demands of Jesus Christ to parishioners. Her total commitment to the poor was an inspiration and a challenge to one's personal faith. Her ability to see Jesus Christ in the poor for whom she provided health care and terminal care stands out. The wounds her sisters bandage are the wounds of Jesus Christ. The dying untouchables to whom they bring love, if only for their last few moments of life, are for them the dying Christ crying out in the agony of abandonment.

The steadfast faith and tender compassion of Mother Teresa and her followers cause countless people to wonder what it is about the person and teachings of Jesus Christ that inspires these women to such devotion and willingness to sacrifice everything to minister to the poorest of the poor. Time and again Mother Teresa repeated the trust she had placed in God who provided whatever she and her sisters needed in order to go where human need exists. This was the case despite the dangers of internal wars, unexpected violence, and governments' heartless rejection of the most vulnerable of their citizens. Hers is the story of trust in God and a steely determination to do something for the otherwise helpless victims and terminally ill "throwaways" of society in all areas of the world to which she could send her sisters.

Mother Teresa's faith is an example of the kind of compassion that is the calling and the challenge of health care providers. Her story is a reminder of the deeper dimensions of the healing profession in which God's Spirit plays a role. In her own writings, she pointed to the poverty of a life without God that is as much a danger as the diseases that she treated.

> The greatest disease in the West today is not TB or leprosy; it is being unwanted, unloved and uncared for. We can cure physical diseases with medicine, but the only cure for loneliness, despair and hopelessness is love. There are many in the world who are dying for a piece of bread but there are many more dying for a little love. The poverty in the West is a different kind of poverty—it is not only a poverty of loneliness but also of spirituality. There's a hunger for love, as there is a hunger for God.[29]

For Mother Teresa, health care was, indeed, in the power of the Spirit.

THEOLOGICAL REFLECTIONS
ON A COMMUNITY OF BELIEVERS

The examples of Cardinal Bernardin, Jean Vanier, and Mother Teresa further illustrate the power of faith to bring hope and healing to vulnerable people and to inspire many of those who have chosen to work in the health care ministry. This ministry is in need of some form of community to sustain the personal faith of health care providers and create a solidarity in which they can find support and encouragement in the difficulties they will inevitably confront in dealing with very sick people. In such a community people can bond in searching for answers to the question of their own significance, dignity and calling. In any ministry that deals with the sick and the handicapped, one must be *trusted by* someone, and at the same time have *faith in* someone. A community of people of faith is likewise helpful not only to continue on individual journeys but also to experience and pass on to others the legacy of faith that enhances health care. Church communities can thus serve as a focus of identity for a community of those who live with and for each other, as is the case with the communities of L'Arche and the Sisters of Charity. Psychologist Eugene Kennedy feels this communitarian support is important to break away from our innate self-centeredness: "I believe the life of the Spirit is something we break into as we break out of ourselves through trying to love more deeply and truly." Developing such a community-centered faith enables us to "throw ourselves away" . . . in the best sense of "being there" for others.[30] In being in each other's company, we are helped in finding out who we really are in the sight of God.

We are convinced that whatever our goals in life may be, faith is the necessary underpinning for leading us in that direction. A person of faith shies away from the nonbeliever's view that "there is no need for faith since one can rely on common sense"—the belief that one can find the answers to life's problems without any reference to God or that what is most ultimate in human existence are the material gains obtained through one's own hard work. This is the proud, independent, self-sufficient person whose material success is a subject of much adulation in today's world. Such adulation is often very shallow. God does not intervene in a theatrical way to dethrone those materialistic individuals from their self-sufficiency. Faith affirms that even the convict on death row is beloved by God. Those who are engaged in prison ministries recognize those convicts as troubled and rejected brothers and sisters of Jesus Christ. Faith affirms that the mentally handicapped person is endowed with a God-given dignity worthy of the best of health care. Faith affirms that the poor, the diseased, the victims of national heartlessness, are also created in the image and likeness of God. Their cries for help and healing are the cries of the Christ tormented on the cross of an evil empire.

When we have integrated faith into our daily living, there comes the realization that we can be both found by and fulfilled by God. This is the highest fulfillment of life to which we can aspire. Once this occurs, and as our faith grows, we may be drawn by the Spirit into daily conversation with God whose guidance we seek through prayer. We may thus experience that unique inner peace found among those who are conscious of God's presence whatever the core of their personal faith.

DISCUSSION QUESTIONS

1. How can we explain the claim that prayer has the power to help people maintain good bodily health? Is there a purely scientific explanation?
2. React to the claim by the noted priest healer Ralph DiOrio on p. 23.
3. Can we share with one another our own understanding of the nature of faith and how we experience faith in our personal lives?
4. Comment on Søren Kierkegaard's view of faith "as a person to whom we commit ourselves irrevocably" and whose "only certitude is trust in the beloved."
5. Comment on Paul Tillich's definition of faith as our "ultimate concern." Do you agree? Is it true that for many in our country their real faith is in money, power, political glory, etc.? Explain.
6. Do you agree with Dietrich Bonhoeffer's understanding of faith as that on which "we stake our lives"? Explain your reaction to this and to Bonhoeffer's assertion that, in faith, "whenever Christ calls us, his call leads us to death."
7. Is there a connection between Karl Rahner's description of faith as a longing for God and Cardinal Bernardin's description of faith as a letting go of our material attachments?
8. Using the example of Jean Vanier, can we say that faith is the inspiration to care for the needy of this world?
9. What does the example of Mother Teresa teach us about the nature of faith?
10. How does the community of believers or, alternately, the communion of saints, teach us about faith in our personal lives?

Chapter 3

Learning Prayer

It is almost a truism that we learn how to pray by praying. Prayer itself is the expression, either vocally or in reverential silence, of the relationship we have with our God. How do we relate to God? How do we get through to God with our needs and concerns? At times, we are similar to the followers of Jesus who asked him: "Lord, teach us to pray" (Luke 11:1).

At other times, we may merit Jesus' laments over the manner of prayer that is unworthy of his Father. Citing Isaiah, he complained: "This people honors me with their lips, but their hearts are far from me" (Matthew 15:8). And in another setting, he criticized those who rattled off prayers "like pagans, for they think that they will be heard because of their many words. Do not be like them, for your Father knows what you need before you ask him" (Matthew 6:7-8). That advice was the prelude to Jesus' teaching his followers the "Our Father." Because of the personal nature of prayer we will attempt in this chapter to describe our own paths in learning how to pray and to add insights that have helped us in praying to the Lord our God. What follows are, therefore, more personal reflections than lessons in steps to take in learning how to pray. We hope that our own struggles in relating to God in prayer may help readers appreciate their potential for growth in their own prayer life.

THEOLOGIAN GEFF'S JOURNEY

The *Imitation of Christ* is very clear on the superiority of knowledge from experience over bookish knowledge. "I would rather feel compunction of heart for my sins than merely know the definition of compunction," Thomas à Kempis declared.[1] Paraphrasing that word of

Is There a God in Health Care?
© 2006 by The Haworth Press, Inc. All rights reserved.
doi:10.1300/5554_03

wisdom: "I would rather be able to pray than to know its definition!" Even if no one can offer an absolute, fit-every-category definition of prayer, most of us know what genuine prayer is and have learned about prayer and how to pray simply by praying. In our Irish Catholic household I was initiated into prayer with the bedtime recitation of a series of "God bless," dutifully heard by Mom, Dad, or Aunt Mae. The list was endless, but was always begun by blessing Mommy and Daddy. At times after an argument or a fight I wanted to eliminate one of my brothers from that litany, but my parents would make me bless them too—my first lesson in forbearance! This was followed by the prayer ditty: "As I lay me down to sleep, I pray the Lord my soul to keep. Watch o'er me this night I pray. Wake me Lord at break of day." Later I found out that some more somber versions of this prayer had the last two lines as "If I should die before I wake, I pray the Lord my soul to take." When someone was sick my blessing prayer was altered to add the words "and make them better."

Only after I had grown well beyond the "terrible twos" and coveted some of the material things others seemed to have in great supply did I begin to add petitions to the Lord to "get me a bicycle," or a "drum," or a "cowboy gun." These "gimme" or requisition prayers were, I soon came to realize, a crapshoot. Sometimes I would get what I prayed for, usually around a birthday or Christmas. Sometimes, the prayer would not produce the desired item. I remember how obnoxiously angry I became when I received the book *Little Men,* instead of a cowboy gun as a Christmas present. Why did God not listen? I had made my wishes known as clearly as possible. Fortunately, I learned early that God could just as easily disappoint me and refuse to grant my most fervent requests. I wondered whether God was angry with me. Why did others get what they wanted? I could not help thinking that maybe I needed to add better pleading or something else to my prayers.

Around the age of six and the beginning of my elementary school education, I learned the "something more" I needed for my requisitions: you do not get something for nothing! I learned the fine art of how to bargain with the Lord. I knew this "great giftgiver" in the sky had power to give us just about anything, including safety from bullies, success in my studies, and the usual list of "needs" that ranged from games to bicycles, to guns, to drums, to boxing gloves, to a cuddly kitten. But I had to offer the Lord some favor on my part to ply his good graces. What if I gave up candy for a period of time? What if I went to church every day? What if I said an extra Rosary? What if I did not fight with my brother? What if I did not get into any fights? What if I did not use foul language as did the other kids in that Irish neighborhood? What if I helped clean the bathroom? Would I then receive what I needed or craved? I felt it was worth a try. Surely God would owe me something for all those good deeds!

Speaking of the Rosary as a bargaining chip, this became the next stage in my learning prayer. It was the great devotion of my Irish parents. It was the most emphasized prayer in our Catholic elementary school. We prayed the Rosary every day and so I quickly learned the Hail Mary, the Our Father, and the Glory Be. The only hitch was to learn and recite the longer and more arduous "Apostles Creed" with which the Rosary began. This was said as we fingered the crucifix around which all the beads were arranged. Just above the crucifix was the first Our Father bead, followed by three Hail Mary beads, and another Our Father bead. Then ten Hail Marys until five decades were completed. The Hail Marys were said while we had the small beads between our finger and thumb; the beads for the Our Fathers were spaced after the first three Hail Marys and after each cluster of ten Hail Marys. At the end of each cluster of Hail Marys we said the Glory Be. By the end of each Rosary we had recited one Apostles Creed, fifty-three Hail Marys, and six Our Fathers. How could God refuse all that, especially since the Rosary was said while we were positioned uncomfortably on our knees? And it took time. It was not convenient. For me, it seemed an irresistible "quid pro quo" offer to God in exchange for almost any favor requested. Sure, there was also a "magic" quality about the Rosary. My mother, for example, said an extra Rosary every day while my brother, Frank was in the army in Korea. No one could ever persuade her that Frank's safe return was due to anything other than the intercession of the Blessed Mother and those Rosaries! Such was her faith. Who is to say that God was not amused or touched enough to guarantee Frank's safe return? Here I am tempted to add: "Don't knock it if you haven't tried it!"

Later when I joined the religious order of the De La Salle Christian Brothers, I was taught how to meditate and how to pray in the spirit of the Founder of the Christian Brothers, Saint John Baptist de La Salle, patron saint of teachers. We could still bargain with God, but now God's refusals were less disappointing, as the Brothers emphasized resignation and acceptance of God's will in our petitions. Saint de La Salle was quoted as having prayed often a strong prayer of resignation: "I adore in all things the guidance of God in my regard."[2] Since we were preparing to take a vow of obedience to go wherever we were to be sent and to do whatever we were assigned, that prayer made a lot of sense. We analyzed the Lord's Prayer and were helped to appreciate Jesus' asking his followers to say "Thy will be done on earth as it is in heaven." Of course, we could still insist that the Lord acquiesce to our own wishes and could pray fervently that *our own will* be done, not without a bit of suspicion or fear of what God might have in store for us. Most of us preferred asking for our daily bread than yielding to God's will, whatever that might be. Our prayers were always prefaced by the exhortation, "Let us remember that we are in the holy presence of God." This was followed by a pause to actually picture ourselves in God's presence. In a way that remembrance was similar to a jolt to our consciousness. God was really present and close to us in a caring, loving way. The thought could fill our young minds with peace and confidence. We also learned to use periods of silence to contemplate God within us in a spiritual presence giving us courage to accept not only who we were but also where God was leading us.

Our public prayers were also channeled outward, away from the inroads of our own selfishness. And so we prayed for the poor, for peace, for the sick, for those recently deceased, for those grieving, for one another, and especially for those in need. The period of meditation directed our thoughts to a sense of the divine presence in the here and now through reflections on Jesus' care of people, especially the children to whom we would devote our lives. Most often the reflections were focused on the service of the poor through religious education, which was the special mission of the Christian Brothers. And so, sometimes bluntly, sometimes subtly, our prayers became less self-centered, not that our self-interests in quiet prayers of petition ever disappeared.

It was not too long after our formation period that the movement began in the Brothers to get rid of those set, stylized morning and evening prayers that represented, not our own feelings, but a rigid seventeenth-century French spirituality. The Brothers were in the process of renewal. Many of us, educated in theology and spirituality, had begun agitating the Brothers' administration to adopt a form of the Breviary, the official prayer of the church.

This shift had a profound effect on my prayer life. The Psalms seemed to capture the moods that were afflicting me in my daily efforts to cope with the demands of teaching high school students while living a rigorous religious life in a community of men. We were taught that these were the prayers Jesus, as a faithful Jew, would pray daily. One could look no further than his despairing cry from the cross, "My God, my God, why have you forsaken me?" (Psalm 22:1) to see how Jesus turned to the Psalms in his moment of anguish. The Lord's Prayer itself was a phrase-by-phrase summary of the principal themes of the Psalms. More than learning how the Psalms were connected with Jesus, the Jewish people, and the daily prayer of the Catholic Church, was the outlet the Psalms provided for praying with all the emotional force that seemed to cover every aspect of life, every demand, every searching for words of praise, every sorrow, every joy. The Psalms became the prayer I turned to in the "downer moments" of community life. Luther himself had recognized the power of the Psalms to bring us into heart to heart communion with the Lord, declaring that once he had begun to pray the Psalms, the other "little devotional prayers" were abandoned in favor of "the strength, the passion, the fire which I find in the Psalter. Anything else tastes too cold and too hard."[3]

What I liked most about the Psalms was the frank way in which they addressed the Lord, the direct, intimate way one speaks to a friend close at hand. The words of love for God should spring from the heart, but are expressed so well in the Psalms that it is easy to make these words become heartfelt words from my own inner depths. In the Psalms I could honestly complain against the hurts of living in community and, in my loneliness, the seeming absence or even abandonment by the God who has promised to take care of me. Here, too, I found the words to proclaim God's fidelity to me and to promise my fidelity to God. Here I could tell the Lord of my moments of depression and my sadness at losing family and friends through death. A Psalm or verses from Psalms were applicable for every mood, every vicissitude of my life. The Psalms offered prayers of thanksgiving, prayers of repentance, prayers of petition, prayers begging for comfort in sorrow, for strength to endure the latest trial, and anger at sins that hurt people. The Psalms helped give me words to express my anguish as well as my joy and to get over the times when my celibate loneliness was overwhelming.

The Psalms were also a source of solace to me when I was passing through my first major crisis as a religious person with vows, the strong sense of dissatisfaction with the community life I was leading. My malaise with living the vowed life had intensified. An overwhelming feeling of loneliness had invaded my efforts to pray and meditate. This and a sense of not being fulfilled in the kind of life to which I had committed myself some twenty years earlier led me finally to request a leave of absence from the Christian Brothers. I also felt unappreciated as a theologian. I had begun to make a name for myself with publications and lectures, but to some in the community this only branded me as too liberal or too out of synch with my own church. At times I felt more at home with my Protestant and Jewish colleagues than with the very Brothers whose life I had shared. It was a time of confusion about what I really wanted to do with my life. My spiritual director was at pains to help me sort out all those conflicting thoughts and emotions. But pray together we did.

At the same time God allowed my future wife, Joan, to enter my life. It soon became clear both to me and my spiritual director that I should seek a dispensation from my vows in order to change my life's direction and marry Joan. My spiritual director assured me that this was God's way of moving me toward other goals that only God at that time could have in mind. My decision to leave the vowed life with the Christian Brothers was bittersweet. I entered a new phase of my life with a certain joy but also with a sadness to leave my lifelong friends in the Brothers. To this day I remain in love with the Christian Brothers with whom I had bonded so closely and shared so much of my life and faith.

I continued to pray the Psalms because the emotions expressed by the Psalmist were so closely aligned with my own feelings and hopes. And yet when my deepest sorrows threatened to overwhelm me and plunge me into the deepest depression, the near death of my daughter, I could only pray the Rosary, that rote prayer that I learned in elementary school and whose words had become so ingrained into my psyche early on in my life. When the crisis had passed I was able again to turn to the Psalms and there I found an even greater peace. When my daughter was near death, I could turn to Psalm 22, verses 1 and 2, and say with more feeling, "My God, my God, why have you forsaken me? Why are you so far from helping me, from the words of my groaning? O my God, I cry by day, but you do not answer; and by night, but find no rest."

I have always been an impatient man. I hate waiting in lines. I hate waiting for answers. I read voraciously and at high velocity just to learn about the characters and their fate as quickly as possible. And I hated waiting for God to come around with the promised help and care and "reward" for my faith. It came as a minor relief from this intensity when my spiritual director asked me to adopt as my own in those moments of impatience, the opening verse of Psalm 62: "For God alone my soul waits in silence; from him comes my salvation." Later he added Psalm 130, verses 5 and 6: "I wait for the Lord, my soul waits, and in his word I hope; my soul waits for the Lord more than those who watch for the morning." Sometimes the waiting still feels similar to an all-nighter. Patience is still an elusive virtue for me.

I liked the direct way the Psalms spoke to the Lord. A rabbi friend of mine once told me that Christians are too formal, rigid, and even cold in our prayers. A believing Jew can use the Psalms or the spirit of the Psalms to argue with God, to remind God of his promises, even, so to speak, to tell God off when everything goes wrong and God seems so remote and absent. "Do you ever argue with a friend, with your parents, with someone you love?" he asked me. Jesus' crying out the opening verse of Psalm 22 seemed to fit well with what my rabbi friend told me. And, yes, thanks to him I could see more clearly how strange my formal prayers to God must have sounded, though I did get my rabbi friend to concede that, sometimes, when our spirits seemed dulled and weary, we needed the formality of set liturgical prayers to help us find words to tell God of our dismay and our personal joys. Is this one of the reasons why we have churches, synagogues, and mosques?

I recalled the rabbi's words during a weekend of retreat and relaxation with some fellow American priests and religious in a picturesque hideaway in the Ardennes Forest of Belgium. We had planned an escape from the intellectual rigors of our courses. We had enjoyed a wonderful happy hour on Friday evening. Over dinner we planned a long morning hike and afternoon sports prior to our Eucharistic celebration. However, that night the skies opened, thunder and lightning seemed to explode all around our chalet, and the windows shook. At around dawn with the skies still pouring a deluvian rain I heard my

Jesuit friend pad across the floor, throw open the window, and shout: "God damn you!" (punctuation just the way I heard it!). He then shut the window, mumbling all the while. The skies began to clear just after breakfast and at around ten o'clock the sun shone in its splendor sending spotlight-like beams through the trees and into the forest. We had a laugh over what this Jesuit priest had done and he joined in the laughter. We all agreed that his less than polite invocation of God's name—or, rather, his reprimanding the weather in God's name—was just what God wanted to hear before returning the sun to brighten our day. After all, did not Jesus rebuke the winds and the waves of an unruly sea (Matthew 8:26)?

Scripture scholar Walter Bruggemann cites the theologian Claus Westermann in concluding that Christian prayer may be "too submissive" when compared to Jewish prayer, where there is at times a vigorous dialog, even a shouting match, filled with protest and demands. We can thus read in Psalm 42, verse 9, these rather blunt words addressed to the Lord: "Why have you forgotten me? Why must I walk about mournfully because the enemy oppresses me?" Bruggemann is convinced that Christians do not pray vigorously because we believe that God is not pictured as responding to shouts. He states the reason for this lack of force in prayers of petition may be due to our fear of upsetting Almighty God, and we lack the right to demand answers from God.[4] Despite these generalizations, some Christians that do cry out and scold God. Every relationship, including God's loving bond with us, his children, or the bond between an earthly father with his children, will from time to time have some strong words spoken.

A more touching story of how a person of faith can speak frankly with God is told by Ann Hallstein, a minister for the United Church of Christ. As a chaplain at Columbia Presbyterian Hospital in New York City she had been summoned to the emergency room where an eight-year-old boy lay dying, victim of a gunshot wound to his head. She had no inkling of what words she could possibly say to the two young women at his bedside, one the mother of the boy, the other her sister. At that moment, their neighbor, a very large black woman, pushed the door open and seemed to fill the room as she grabbed the two young women and held them tightly. She began to comfort them, hushing their tears and calling them her babies although she was only their neighbor. Ann Hallstein recalled her words:

> And then, in a commanding voice full of authority, she ordered Jesus to come into the room "right this minute, come in here, Jesus, my babies need you, and they need you *now*, I don't mean later, I don't mean in ten minutes, I mean NOW! Get down here! Come into this room and comfort these babies! Jesus, Jesus, get in here now, there's nothing anyone can do but *you*."[5]

Hallstein then felt a calm come over everyone as this neighbor held the young women in her arms and rocked them. Hallstein also put her arms around all of them and together they swayed back and forth. They had lost any sense of time or place and felt only the love of this neighbor and the love of God her presence and words had brought into that emergency room. Hallstein's reflections on that experience are worth repeating:

> She soon left, but the palpable sense of love and comfort remained long after the few minutes of her presence. Prayer? You bet—the most immediate, most effective and most powerful I've seen. I could tell that what fueled her, what "made it happen" was that she was fully present, totally open and full of both love and faith. She was *there,* she summoned God there, and it was her presence that invoked the healing needed at that moment.[6]

I often see this kind of faith when I attend healing services. I find it gratifying to see how the prayers of a person of faith can reach the level wherein speaking one's mind to the Lord in spontaneity becomes natural. I am reassured when I observe the confidence that emanates from the prayers of those who are so obviously intimate with the Lord. Many of the saints were known for their confident persistence. When I became a spiritual director for the De La Salle Christian Brothers, I spoke often about the need to develop a sense of God's presence and a personal prayer life that leads to intimacy with God. Realistically, we were all at different levels of awareness of the divine presence and of familiarity with God. Not all of us were satisfied with the quality of our prayers—the quantity was no problem; our structured prayers at regular hours took care of that! Yet, to believe the mystics and to take lessons from the lives of the saints such intimacy was exactly where God would lead us if we dare follow. I taught the Psalms, hoping that as they prayed the Breviary, a love for these prayers of the Bible might take hold in the hearts of those young Brothers just beginning their religious lives. Whatever has developed in me or in the Brothers whose lives I shared for over twenty years is impossible to depict adequately. Their two great gifts to me, which were received in turn from Saint John Baptist de La Salle, were that sense of God's presence through the continual reminder, "Let us remember that we are in the holy presence of God," and the invocation that became a sign of our identity as Christian Brothers, "Live, Jesus, in our hearts! Forever!"

One effect of the practice of the presence of God and praying the Psalms was the strong need that came over both Bill and me to meditate on selected passages of the scriptures. This has become a daily practice, similar to beginning the day with breakfast. I would read a text, sometimes with a commentary, such as one finds in the *Daily Texts,* published by the Moravian Church, or made available in the *Daily Word* that we receive each month. We take these texts as a word from the Lord whose meaning we could ponder for an hour or so in peaceful silence away from the noise of our daily lives and the treadmill existence at our places of work. We have taken to heart what Dietrich Bonhoeffer had once urged on his seminarians, namely, the practice of daily meditation as a strength in their unique mission to subvert Nazism through their church ministry. He told them, many of whom had been drafted into the German Army and sent to fight on the Russian front, that this meditative prayer

> was the focal point of everything which brings inward and outward order into [their] life. . . . Meditation gives our life something like constancy; it keeps the link with our previous life, from baptism to confirmation, to ordination. It keeps us in the saving fellowship of the community, the brethren, our spiritual home . . . It is a source of peace, of patience, and of joy . . .[7]

Of course, our own time out for meditation still begins with the call for us to remember that we are in the holy presence of God no matter where we are settled for meditation, whether in a corner of the house, at the university chapel, in the medical offices, or in the open air during a long early morning walk.

Over my many years as a religious with vows, as a married man with children, and as a teacher and spiritual director, whether praying with young children or older adults, I have learned that there are no set ways in which individuals pray to the one we acknowledge as our God and Lord. Indeed, the unsophisticated prayers of little children have a special charm. I find the prayers of sick children to be even more heartwarming because of their innocence and vulnerability. I understand why Jesus could tell the apostles to get out of the way so the little children could come to him. Before taking my then terminally ill daughter to the healer priest Reverend Ralph DiOrio, I had heard that his most heartbreaking moments occurred when, with the little children on whom he placed his hands and prayed for their healing, his pleas with the Lord seemed to have no effect on their physical illness. I later experienced that beyond every physical cure is the more important spiritual healing that is a prelude to our eternal life with the Lord.

In helping the mother of one of my students who had asked me to meet and speak with her during her terminal illness, our prayers together were always spontaneous whether at the beginning of our conversations or, as we ended our sessions, after having spent an hour discussing theology and religion, particularly about death and resurrection. We prayed as the Spirit moved us over what we had shared and over her concerns and anxiety, facing death as she was. During some of the worst periods of my daughter's illness, a local pastor of a bible church would phone me and pray with me for my daughter and my family over the telephone. His words were beautiful and close to those biblical texts that offered both consolation and confidence in God's healing power. St. Paul says it well. The Holy Spirit prays through our spirit giving us the words and the strength to pour out our hearts to the Lord (Romans 8:26-27). There was an indefinable power in those prayers that had sprung from the heart with words whose beauty and force seemed completely God-given.

Ways to pray are endless. Teresa of Avila, for example, called prayer a friendly conversation with God. She began her prayer time by audibly reciting the Lord's Prayer, followed by gradually sliding into mental prayer which, for her, was the gateway to a deep contemplative union with God. Gazing upon an icon of Jesus helped her to focus on Jesus, the one to whom she prayed. Teresa believed that we should never tire of the "Our Father" as it was the starting point for her path to mystical communion with God.[8]

Just as there are a number of different types of prayer, there are also those inevitable "dry times" when prayer seems far away from our hearts. Even the saints were once beginners in prayer, and they had many differing approaches to God. St. Francis, for one, preferred prayers of thanksgiving and praise as the more effective way to pray than prayers of petition. Francis had the unique grace of being able to recognize God in all creation and at all times and all places. Sometimes he turned to prayer, and at other times he turned *into* prayer. He lived and never let go of God's constant presence.

But Francis was also conscious of the need for people to pray for one another's needs. Such prayers of intercession bring us back to those moments when in our childhood we called down God's blessings and healings on those who were part of our infantile litany of concern. Most of us began to pray this way. As we grow older, our awareness of our dependence on one another is never so intense as in those moments when we experience the need of having people pray for us and for our intentions. Dietrich Bonhoeffer said it very well in *Life Together,* a spiritual classic on Christian Community: "A Christian community either lives by the intercessory prayers of its members for one another or the community will be destroyed."[9] Bonhoeffer knew that to pray for others achieved what was often considered nearly impossible among people cast together by all the unpredictable directions one's life could take. In prayers of intercession, enemies could be forgiven, burdens lightened, and sorrows alleviated. In prison he was not ashamed to ask his friend, Eberhard Bethge, to promise that they

> remain faithful in interceding for each other . . . And if it should be decided that we are not to meet again, let us remember each other to the end in thankfulness and forgiveness, and may God grant us that one day we may stand before [God] praying for each other and joining in praise and thankfulness.[10]

Theologian Karl Rahner warns Christians not to take their promises of intercessory prayer as something merely perfunctory, "fossil fragments of from times gone by," when we could easily say to another "I'll pray for you," and then allow the promise to die a death of neglect.[11] Praying with and for others is the lifeblood of compassion within the Christian community. Such prayers open up the community to other worlds where God's people cry out in their distress to their unknown brothers and sisters bound together in a communion of persons created in God's image and likeness and, whether friend or enemy, brother and sister to Jesus Christ.

I experienced a striking example of the power of intercessory prayer in the late 1970s when a close friend, Tom Ryan, a former Christian Brother, lay dying of leukemia. He had been in the hospital less than a week and already the hemorrhaging had begun. He was not expected to live much longer. Tom and Eileen had a five-year-old daughter at home. There seemed to be no hope that Tom would recover. Eileen had to be home in the nights tending to young Eileen but with the understanding that the hospital would phone her if Tom took a turn for the worse. A prayer group, knowing the Ryans, promised to say special prayers for Tom. They did so at 9:00 p.m. on a night when, to the doctors, Tom seemed to be sinking. At 6:00 the next morning Eileen heard the phone ringing. She had only one thought: Tom was either dead or expected to die that day, and she was being summoned to the hospital. She answered the phone and heard Tom's voice telling her that he felt much better and that the previous evening at 9:00 he could feel a surge of strength. The medicine had kicked in. Later, Eileen told him that at the precise moment of those intercessory prayers his condition improved. Tom went into spontaneous remission which lasted for a precious year of life in which he could put his affairs in order and help his family and friends adjust to his passing into everlasting life. It was a year of grace and, as with most physical healings, a welcome reprieve from a death that would otherwise have been too sudden for his family to bear.

Finally, to pray for one another is an essential part of most worship services. Invoking our God and Lord on behalf of others is not only a confession of our faith in the power and providence of God but also an outreach of compassion for one another. Our communion in faith with those whom God has given us to love and care for, whether neighbors near to us within a parish or "neighbors" in distant lands but bound to us through our common humanity, is never so intense as during those moments when we speak their names to the Lord asking for their healing and the fulfillment of their needs. Through intercessory prayer, we can reach the level that both Luther and Dietrich Bonhoeffer have proclaimed as "being transformed into one another through love," and where we are "bound to reach the point where the want, infirmities, and sins of [our]neighbor afflict [us] as if they were [our] own . . ."[12]

Whatever the form or the words it assumes, prayer is fundamentally the offering of our hearts to God and when we are two or three praying together, it is also the offering of our hearts to one another. When Doctor Bill speaks of prayer as an integral part of the healing process, he is describing not only the lifting up of our spirits to acknowledge the power of God over our life and death but also the effect on our physical and spiritual well-being of the communion of one person with another in the presence of God. Prayer is not the addition of another tool in the arsenal of healing that doctors tap into; the prayers offered within the practice of the healing professions place us in the presence of the source of well-being whether physical, emotional, or spiritual.

DOCTOR BILL'S JOURNEY
TO A DEEPENED FAITH IN PRAYER

Similar to Geff, my prayer life began at bedtime when my mother taught me to say my "God bless" on all family persons. This would include grandparents, aunts, uncles, and Mommy and Daddy. A few years later, when old enough for Sunday school, my father, mother, and I would go to church together. At some point before the sermon and Eucharist, the children were excused and hurried off to religion classes until the end of the service when we were claimed before starting for home. I remember a small pin, shaped like a shield, that had the number of years of good attendance inscribed on it for all to see. But I must confess that I, along with most of us in that captive audience of children, did not get much out of the Sunday school; we would rather be outside playing. This church was an Episcopal church down the street from our house. After my father died, we moved to my grandparents' home on a busy main street five miles away. It was the time of World War II and a Presbyterian church, just across the street and a short walk away, became our new house for worship. The fact that gasoline was rationed made a short walk to church all the more attractive.

When I was thirteen years old, by prayers and good fortune—details to follow later in this book—I was fortunate to receive a financial scholarship enabling me to attend Newark Academy, an outstanding private day school. The daily morning chapel service lingers with me as a strong memory of my time at that school. The service included a brief scripture reading, announcements, and one of the grand old hymns. To this day I still love singing these hymns among which were the lyrical melodies of "Holy, Holy, Holy" and "Fling Out the Banner." Tears filled my eyes whenever we sang, "Faith of our fathers, holy faith. We will be true to thee till death," because it brought home to me the memories of my father's love and the sorrow over his recent death.

In March 1944, my senior year at Newark Academy, I was accepted for appointment to the United States Merchant Marine Academy at Kings Point, Long Island. I had to take early exams to receive the credit from the Newark Academy to begin my plebe training. This forced me to miss the June graduation. By that time, I had completed three months of hurry-up training and was headed for a ship on the West Coast that was being readied for a trip to Saipan in the Pacific theater. All five holds in the ship were loaded with drums of 100 octane gasoline. Army trucks and other army paraphernalia were lashed to the deck leaving only a few inches of freeboard space. Saipan was destined to be a site for B-29 bombers whose mission was to begin their raids on the Japanese empire.

By that time, my mother had introduced me to the *Daily Word,* a publication that provided a spiritual message for each day. The readings helped me appreciate the power of faith in speaking of our needs to God. Then as now, this small booklet has helped me to live each day in the faith that God is always present and guiding us. The custom of reading the *Daily Word* is one of the most precious and lasting gifts of my mother to me in my own spiritual formation. My *Daily Word* was always with me, and each day I knew my mother and her eighteen-year-old son would be reading the same message. A sense of closeness was felt by this practice. She had no idea where we were in the Pacific as was the case during the war for all of us servicemen. The mail was censored anyway; this was serious business. One hundred and forty-two fellow merchant marine cadets were lost in enemy actions when their ships were torpedoed, hit by surface enemy ships, or attacked by kamikaze planes.

On returning home safely, I learned that my mother had also prayed for me during my stint in the Pacific during World War II. Since the mail was heavily censored, families had no idea where their sons were. I remember opening a package from my mother containing winter underwear and receiving a pipe from my uncle. Little did my mother realize her son was aboard a ship docked at Saipan where the temperature was ninety-five degrees. Being a nonsmoker, I choked after one puff from the pipe and threw it in the trash. It was a time when Bing Crosby was singing, "I'm dreaming of a white Christmas," while Japanese bombers were overhead. It was a strange time, that hot Christmas in 1944, made bearable by the knowledge that my mother was praying for my safe return.

In March 1946, our section graduated from the Merchant Marine Academy and we received our Navy commissions signed by the Secretary of the Navy, James Forrestal, and also a third mate's license issued by the United States Coast Guard. I was promptly assigned to a troopship that carried 1,500 German and Italian prisoners of war home to Bremerhaven, Germany, and United States troops returning home to New York. By now the war had just ended and I was in charge of the 12 to 4 watch as the third officer. One episode I will always remember to reinforce my growing conviction that God answered my prayers occurred during my watch while we were sailing in a deep fog in the English Channel at night. The ship, having no radar, was forced to proceed at "slow ahead" because of the limited vision. The ship's whistle was sounded at regular intervals, warning any nearby ships or fishing boats that we were underway and to get out of our path. In these circumstances, there is always a lookout at the bow who would also ring the ship's bell at frequent intervals, much as in the older days of sailing ships. To add to the complexity was the fact that mines had become loose and the Channel minesweepers had not fully picked them up.

Even more important for me was the fact that some of the navigation buoys were also missing. We had relied on these to determine the course of the vessel since these were identified by their location in the chart room. Compounding this problem the captain was ill and so only the helmsman and I were on the bridge. Everything seemed to be all right so long as the buoys were present to help whenever there was an alteration of the ship's course. Knowing the speed and time and direction in which the ship was moving, I noted that a buoy which should have been bobbing in the water was not in its expected location. With a sinking feeling and knowing there were over 1,500 people onboard, I altered course, assuming that the buoy was present in its proper place. If ever there was a time for me to call upon the Lord to protect me and those 1,500 people whose lives were dependent on our judgment, that was it!

With a sign of relief the next buoy was there and in its proper place! The rest of the evening was fortunately uneventful. Looking back over my career in medicine, I do not remember a greater sense of responsibility or a moment when I was called to place my complete trust in the Lord's protection. This nineteen-year-old learned to call on God's guidance and to be assured that God does answer prayers.

Troopships seemed to become my middle name, because the Navy called me to active duty between 1955 and 1957, just after I had finished medical school and put in one year of medical internship. This time I was assigned as the ship's medical officer to a troopship carrying 2,500 men, women, and children, all of whom had escaped from countries behind the Iron Curtain. We had a small cadre of officers, a full staff of nurses and corpsmen, and other shipboard Navy personnel. The field of general medicine on that trip, which consisted mainly of endless cases of sea sickness, was amplified by twenty-six dental extractions due to abscessed teeth among those coming to the States and sewing back the remainder of a dog's tail damaged in rough weather. A new zest for medical practice appeared by my becoming an amateur dentist and vet. The "hospital" was equipped for almost anything from orthopedic surgery to dental surgery. Having been exposed to only six weeks of surgical training as a medical intern, I hardly felt competent to handle a surgical emergency at any time, but even less so on a rolling ship. This possibility, or rather the evasion of this possibility, was high on my prayer list. My prayers were again answered!

Since the end of my times at sea I have had frequent occasions to look back and reflect upon the sixty-four Atlantic, four Pacific, and four Caribbean crossings that I made so many years ago. A special emotional feeling of peace is present when one is at sea, even though one is always happy to get back on land. God shows the divine majesty during times of mighty storms with waves breaking over the bridge as well as during the times when God calmly speaks to us through beautiful sunrises or magnificent sunsets. At other times I have emblazoned in my memory God's palpable closeness while standing alone on the flying bridge and being awestruck by the glory of a sky full of stars and a sea so calm that the stars were reflected on the water similar to a mirror. That experience helped me appreciate Brother Lawrence's classic book on practicing the presence of God.[13] The comfort of knowing that God is present to and even within us at all times can be an anchor in our spiritual journey, knowing that God has a divine plan for each of us and, whatever our circumstances may be, God will never leave us.

Over time I found that prayer enables us to listen for God's guidance. Many of the readings I have taken to heart only reinforced those earlier awakenings to God's presence and to the inexpressible calm that can enter my heart through prayer. Reverend David Read, Pastor Emeritus of the Madison Avenue Presbyterian Church, wrote an article in *The Living Pulpit* that could serve as a cautionary tale as Geff and I write about prayer: "So You're Preaching on Prayer? God Help You." I hope God is helping us in this endeavor. Read believes that, if we are to talk to others about prayer, we certainly have to incorporate prayer in our daily lives as well. In a similar vein, physicians who stress the need for daily physical exercise would soon lose their integrity should they do none at all. Read goes on to say it does not matter how close we may feel to God or what the quality of the prayer may be. We should "just do it!"[14] As did Read, I discovered that I needed to be quiet in the presence of God, to shut out all the extraneous noise, and to allow the Spirit to guide me in my prayers.

The late Sister Miriam Murphy, a dear friend and my spiritual advisor for twenty years, often remarked that the goal of the mature Christian life is to enter into a communion with God. As we mature, we move from a stage of *communication* with God to one of *communion* with God. For her, as for me, this stage is where Jesus Christ becomes a living presence and empowering force with us. Prayer becomes action as God's outreach to those in need emanates from being in daily communion with the divine presence. Those prayers are incessant in God's inspiring us to help those who are suffering. In this way and led by God's spirit, we become a channel of grace and divine providence for others.[15] For those who are learning to pray, it is not necessary to employ "the correct words." God listens to us regardless of our mode of praying. As we grow in the awareness that God is present within us we begin to speak to God as a friend. St. Paul is incessant in his observation that God's Spirit will speak through us and the words will be under the guidance of the same spirit (Romans 8:26-28).

Even with the earlier experiences of God's presence and the realization that, indeed, God did answer my prayers, my increased awareness of God's presence in my life did not fully enter my heart until later in my medical career. As have all of the people who are a part of my life, I had to undergo periods of unexpected suffering in order to appreciate more fully God's designs on me in my vocation as a husband, father, and skilled physician. Looking back on the crisis moments in my life, I can now see the suffering as additional gifts of God's grace.

My journey, as in the case of so many other individuals I have come to know as my friends and patients, began in earnest following a time of personal brokenness. Two such painful growth periods brought me unwittingly closer to God. The first was the death of my father from liver failure, most likely due to hepatitis C contracted during World War I at the time of the flu epidemic of 1918. This occurred just three days before his forty-second birthday and my twelfth birthday; we both were born on June sixth. It was heartbreaking for both my mother and me to see that handsome, robust man fade away, to hear his semicomatose groans at night, and to view his ever-increasing jaundice. We felt helpless and devastated watching him slowly die before our eyes. His only survivors were my mother, an elementary school teacher, and me. Being "broken" left both my mother and me with few options. We became completely "open" with each other and with the Lord. The tragedy forced us to reaffirm our belief totally in God's love and the divine plan for us. This was a time of a strong bonding between the two of us. We could go on only with such trust in each other and in the Lord despite the loss of the one who was dearest to us. Our funds were very limited; I remember the day my mother and I celebrated her raise in salary to $4,000 a year! Many years later I learned that my mother had pawned her engagement ring following my father's death so that she could purchase a train set for our first Christmas without him. What a sacrifice for her! Fortunately she was able to recover the ring soon afterward.

Likewise, this was a time of realizing that God really did hear our prayers—prayers that thanked God for looking after us and for providing for us. We began reading the *Daily Word,* a nondenominational Christian pamphlet, that would serve me well during my years of naval service. Its incorporation of scripture texts and inspirational comments in its everyday messages became a source of affirmation to us in those uncertain times. My mother and I turned to God for our support and guidance through these daily texts. In an uncanny way those readings for each day of the year seemed to speak almost intuitively to whatever was our specific concern for that time. My mother continued to read the *Daily Word* religiously for the rest of her life. I have continually read these texts since the age of thirteen, but in recent years I have supplemented this booklet with other spiritual works, and since 1980 I have kept a spiritual journal as well.

The beautiful messages proclaimed in various ways and addressed to different events in our lives, seemed to focus upon the word *affirmation*. Although we had very little in the form of financial resources, thanking God in advance for God's blessings in the past, for those of the present, and trusting in God's grace for potential needs in the future, helped us live each day in the faith that God was always present and guiding us. God's presence appeared now to manifest the divine love for us in virtually all aspects of our lives. The format of our prayers at that time, which has continued for me even to this day, consists of prayers of affirmation: trusting and thanking God for already hearing them and acting upon them according to the divine plan. Many of these prayers concerned her life and work and many concerned her son (me) and my education. She soon became an author of the Ginn & Co. Basic Reading Series and was promoted to elementary supervisor for the five Orange, New Jersey, public schools. She was well into finishing her PhD in education at Montclair Teacher's College when she died from a series of small strokes.

My mother's philosophy of life and survival was to thank God for providing for all our needs. Always affirmative when it came to prayer, she thanked God in advance for her promotion in the school system—she had started out as a substitute teacher in those early days with little hope of promotion. Another example of her trusting, affirmative prayer was her requests to the Lord for help in my education. She again thanked God even before any concrete answer to this petition had been received. She trusted God's response would be positive even before the answer came in the form of my obtaining a full scholarship to Newark Academy. The same held for my being accepted at Princeton University and finally in my obtaining free education at Columbia Medical School.

Of course, how God answers prayers was and still remains a mystery of the subtle ways of God's interventions. My acceptance at Columbia is a story in itself. Dr. Bilhuber and his wife, Belle, lived down the street from us. They had no children, but they became a courtesy "uncle" and "aunt" to me. We frequently greeted each other whenever I walked my dog by their house. He was a successful pharmaceutical manufacturer and allowed five of my friends to transform the top floor of his garage into the "Sandow Weightlifting Club," named after the immortal Eugene Sandow who lived in Austria at the turn of the century. He was an old-fashioned weightlifter who sported a handlebar mustache. He wore a leopard outfit and used a barbell with the globe-shaped weights at each end. It must have been quite a sight to see: five skinny fourteen- to sixteen-year-olds lifting weights and hoping to be instantly transformed into Mr. America. "Uncle" Ernie had also graduated from Princeton and earned his doctorate in pharmacology at Columbia. He had followed my journey over the years, and so when I was accepted to the College of Physicians and Surgeons, I was pleasantly shocked when one day he said, "Bill, I want to pay for your medical school, and I don't want you to pay me back!" I did repay him after being in practice a few years.

At the time we had been wondering how we could afford four years of medical education on my mother's salary as a teacher. Here again, she thanked God ahead of time for helping me to finance my medical education at Columbia. When my benefactor offered to pay for my education my mother was convinced that this act of benevolence was the result of her prayers of affirmation. I have described some of her prayers and tactics with the Lord in a previous book, under the heading, "Love Letters to God."[16] She would often remark: "The more you thank God for your blessings, the more blessings will come your way." In my case this has been so true.

Through the faith that God and all the influences God provided in my life, all the prayers were answered even though *there was no obvious answer in sight*—all done with trust in God's providence and plan. All prayers were accompanied with thanks for God's response, realizing that it would be God's answer, and not necessarily one we might envision. My entire life of faith, as well as my mother's, has been based upon this thankfulness for God's loving plan. The mechanism involved was to write an actual letter to God concerning the need or concern at hand, to thank God for handling it according to the divine will. The letter was signed and placed into an envelope, which was sealed. The date and the word "Personal" were written on the envelope. This "love letter to God" was then placed in the Bible, or in a desk drawer out of sight, an action that was tantamount to turning it over to God. Months or years later, the letter might be discovered while rummaging through the desk drawer and when opened, the prayer was either answered, or when different, revealed that God's plan was better in hindsight than what was hoped for originally. This serves as a reminder that God loves us, and prayers are answered but according to *God's plan* and in God's time and not necessarily ours. This is a powerful way to allow us to experience a very personal encounter with God. I have had dozens of patients who also employ this method successfully for their own concerns over the years.

A second turbulent time in my life shattered any complacency that I may have built up—my divorce. It was a time of the so-called midlife crisis of the late 1970s and early 1980s. The nation was being awakened by the birth of a strong feminist movement. After nearly twenty years of marriage my wife informed me that she did not want to be the wife of a doctor any longer. I was totally unprepared for this shock as I thought we had enjoyed a very good relationship over the years. Not the least of my sadness was the fact that three wonderful teenagers were caught in this personal tragedy. They were understandably upset with this sudden and unexpected turn of events. Thankfully, with God's help, self-forgiveness and forgiveness of one another prevailed. The children continued to be bathed in love. Slowly I came to realize that both parents must share in the responsibility for the dissolution of any marriage. Back then my wife's announcement took me completely by surprise. In the months that followed I would wake up around 3:00 a.m. and go for a run around the block. With tears running down my cheeks I somehow found the words to "thank" God for this catastrophe. The prayers of affirmation and thanksgiving that, thanks to my mother, had been ingrained in my psyche kicked in and offered me the only consolation I could find. I knew in my heart that God would never abandon us. I still trusted in the divine plan for all of us. God was there for us all, and our children have remained close to our hearts. They are all happily married now with children of their own.

Well, God did not abandon me or my children. However, for the next four years I was in my "desert experience." This was a time for great spiritual transformation: many retreats, prayers, and I read numerous books on healing. Finally, one of the answers to my prayers came in the form of a divine intervention that brought me a spiritual guide. Her name was Sister Miriam Murphy, who at that time was a visiting fellow at the Princeton Theological Seminary. Our spiritual relationship was the direct outcome of a routine office visit during that dark time in my personal life. After taking care of her physical complaint, we somehow started to talk about meditation and prayer. This led to her becoming my spiritual director during the next twenty years. Nearly every Monday at noon we would have a small lunch, discuss any of life's complicating events, and pray for each other's needs. I would usually leave with a book, an article, or notice of a retreat on inner healing. This became for me a "divine encounter." In my faith I believe that the Lord had arranged for this wise and faith-filled educator to walk into my life and become a wonderful resource of strength and guidance. She helped me to enter an even deeper spiritual level and see the hand of God even in the sorrowing event of my divorce. Under her direction my prayer life was nurtured and my healing ministry was given more meaning. No human persuasion can ever convince me that our first encounter was purely accidental. Our relationship continued for the next twenty-two years and was ended only by her death a few years ago.

My new but sad journey opened the door for God's grace and inner healing as well as a time of transformation from the persona of a trained scientist to one cognizant of the power of God within me as well as within those others who would make demands on my time and energies. One of the problems with being a scientist—in my case a physician—was the inability to become vulnerable when dealing with patients. Sister Miriam sent me to the Annual Charismatic Conference at Notre Dame. About 10,000 people were present: priests, monsignors, bishops, and laity all praising God with their arms extended to heaven. It reminded me of a Pentecostal revival rather than a gathering of members of the hierarchy and laity of the Catholic Church. It helped me to raise my arms in praise of God. This was something new for me. I had always thought that Catholics were just as zipped up and guarded as the Episcopalians about showing emotions during a church service. If those attending this conference felt so uninhibited in praising God, I should feel free to drop some of my own inhibitions and praise the Lord with them. The experience helped me get more closely in touch with my own emotions and begin to lose some of that scientific complacency and emotional distance from my patients.

Another turn in the emotional side of my prayer life came through a patient of mine, Reverend Jesse Owens of the Nassau Christian Center in Princeton. This church represented a spirit-filled Assembly of God tradition. The entire church from the walls to the ceiling seemed to sway with vibrant songs of praise every Sunday evening. Strangers were welcomed with a hug. Their way of worship was contagious: powerful sermons and equally joyous songs sending praises up to God. The Holy Spirit's presence was palpable! It was natural to be caught up in the rhapsodic atmosphere of such a worship. I was pleasantly surprised during one of those services to recognize our Episcopal rector taking part in one of the Spirit-filled services.

Jesse and I often prayed during his routine office visits. His wife, Kay, was also a very God-loving and deeply Christian believer. One time, during the early days of my being alone, Jesse must have spotted me sitting in the back of the church. At the conclusion of his service and just as I had crossed the street in front of the church, he left people standing at the church door and ran after me. He told me that if I were going to be alone for Thanksgiving, he wanted me to join his family for dinner. His kind acts in the midst of my bouts with loneliness will always be remembered. A few years later, he answered a call to the foreign missions and left Princeton to start up a number of new churches in several third world countries. On more than one occasion, on a Sunday evening, a member of his church would phone to make sure I was okay. This thoughtfulness helped me never to lose sight of just how good people can be and how important it is to be a member of a community of believers.

It seemed that everyone in town was praying for me and the children, all denominations. A beloved patient, Sister Carmody, having moved to Kenwood, a retirement home for Sisters of the Sacred Heart, placed my name on the daily prayer list where all the "saints" living there took part. She would write often, and would reassure me that I was being showered by prayer every day. The stories could go on but the power of prayer was there on all occasions leading to my inner healing. Knowing of their intercessions reinforced my belief in prayer and its relationship to healing and told me, better than anything I had experienced before, that God does have a plan for each of us. I was called to be more than a skilled scientist or a medical mechanic. I was called to be a physician healer and now a disciple of Christ as well.

One event that will remain in my memory occurred when I was on a retreat in Florida given by a retired Methodist bishop. The retreat was dedicated to prayer and healing. Each participant who so desired would sit on a chair in the middle of a prayer circle and one by one would be the recipient of prayers for healing with the laying on of hands. While I was being prayed for, the bishop, after placing his hand on me, whispered into my ear, "Please pray for me too." This came at the time as a revelation since somehow I had thought that the clergy were well served by prayers at all times and were the givers of healing with little need for the healing I was then experiencing. Having come to know many clergymen since then and having shared prayers and reflections with these dedicated ministers, I have appreciated even more the work they do for the Lord despite the failings that seem to be our human lot on earth and the emotional needs that they too must cope with.

As my personal healing progressed so too did the new beginning in my life's journey. I experienced a new avocation, that of lecturing on prayer, being used as adjunct to the practice of medicine, and to do some writing on the subject. Toward the end of my "desert time," I met my wife, Aline. She is a real spiritual partner who has brought joy and caring into my life. We have been married for twenty years as of this writing. The "desert time" I experienced had many advantages. It became a time for reflection, inner healing, and, for me, a time to see how prayer has such a power to aid us in the healing process. Without having been broken, so to speak, and led into the "desert" coping with personal hurt and loneliness, my lectures on prayer and the practice of medicine and my writing on the importance of prayer would not have had as much impact on those who have been helped by my own experience.

We not often receive confirmation that something we may have said or done has helped bring about a healing in another. Not long ago, however, I did receive a letter from a sixty-three-year-old patient who was a survivor of a series of cardiac problems. Charles had been invited by a Methodist minister who had read my earlier book, *A Physician's Witness to the Power of Shared Prayer,* and asked Charles to tell his story. The minister knew that my patient had received many prayers offered both with and for him. I had sent him to the Robert Wood Johnson Medical Center for further procedures, but not before we had prayed with the affirmation that he would, with God's healing power and his own faith conjoined, experience a full and complete recovery.

Praying with and for him also brought one of the attending nurses back to her Roman Catholic Church after many years away. She had seen up close what faith can do in healing. My patient's words touched my heart: "After all these years this is still an emotional story for me to tell. But I felt an obligation to share the story and to be a witness—a patient's witness to the power of prayer. Many people came up to me after the service and thanked me for the story. Two physicians came to the talk: one, a retired psychiatrist, was a believer, and the other, was doubtful but unable to deny the story." Afterward, he made this remark to a fellow parishioner. "You never know how far-reaching the message can go when you are God's messenger." He closed by thanking me for being his physician and for "helping me recover my faith." Indeed, sometimes our prayers for one another never seem to bring the palpable results we like to see, perhaps in a throwback to our empirical bent. Testimonies such as that of my patient help me continue to trust in the Lord and to be grateful for the relationships that bind me with my patients as we express our common faith in the Lord, the ultimate healer.

By the end of that "dark night" or what I have called my "desert time," I had been able to see more clearly just how affirmative prayer plays a role even when times can be very bleak. My spiritual journey keeps being enhanced through God's grace. I became professed as a Third Order Franciscan. I have been praying with and for my patients, giving lectures on prayer and healing. In addition, I have written two books on prayer and the practice of medicine and, with God's help, graduated with highest honors at age seventy-four from La Salle's Graduate School of Religious Studies with a master's degree in theological and pastoral studies. I am told I was the oldest duffer ever to graduate from this department. Finally, at La Salle I had the good fortune to meet and work with Geff Kelly. The Lord has been good to me and I keep thanking him for all the blessings, some hidden in what looked like tragedy and sorrow.

The journey continues. My daily time with the Lord begins in the morning with listening for fifteen or twenty minutes, followed by reading selected literature and engaging in silent prayer. I keep a journal. This enables me to take God's presence from the time devoted to meditation into the busy day. In a way I have become a practicing contemplative, at least I have tried to maintain the presence of God throughout the day as best as I am able. I once thought I was walking in darkness. God's care led me back to the words of Jesus: "I am the light of the world. Whoever follows me will never walk in darkness, but will have the light of life" (John 8:12). Prayer for me is that light in the darkness which always threatens to engulf us.

DISCUSSION QUESTIONS

1. Comment on the assertion that we learn to pray by praying.
2. Why are the "gimme" or requisition prayers often considered by theologians and spiritual writers to be a "crapshoot"?
3. Comment on the "bargain with God" kind of prayer. Have you ever engaged in this kind of prayer with any success?
4. What are the special benefits of praying the Psalms? Comment on Luther's claim that he found "the strength, the passion, the fire" in the Jewish Book of Psalms.
5. Is it possible or even respectable to cry out in a "scolding" way to God or even complain to God in prayer?
6. Why are intercessory prayers so important in health care? Why does Rahner warn us not to take promises of intercessory prayers lightly?
7. How can a positive answer to our prayers strengthen both our faith and prayer life?
8. What is meditation? Contemplation? How can we integrate meditation into our daily lives in health care? What are the benefits?
9. What do you think of the practice of thanking God ahead of time in prayer, that is, to pray in anticipation of God's granting our petition?
10. How has prayer helped us or how *can* prayer help us survive the trials and sufferings of life?

Chapter 4

Jesus' Healing Ministry and Sufferings Related to Personal Experiences

GOD AS THE "FATHER"

The God whom we have come to know in our daily lives, whether in a cardiologist's medical practice or a theologian's encounter with his students, is more akin to the God whom Jesus called Father and to Jesus himself who, as the scriptural testimony proclaimed, made common cause with the sick and social outcasts of his society. Peter preached in Acts that Jesus "went about doing good" (Acts 10:38). Jesus had nothing to do with the Oriental potentate type of deity that could be extrapolated from ritual practices of some cultures or the distorted images of a God of violence and wrath in narrow readings of certain scriptural texts. Before his execution at the hands of brutal SS camp guards, Dietrich Bonhoeffer wrote that Christian faith had to reject these false images of God. God was not a *deus ex machina* dropping to earth at the opportune moment to prop up human weakness and solve problems too difficult for ordinary humans; nor was God a fallback, abstract deity invoked to fill in the gaps when human intellection failed to offer adequate explanations for the tragedies that beset human life. Instead, he offered this portrait of his God, father to Jesus Christ:

> God lets God be pushed out of the world on to the cross. God is weak and powerless in the world, and that is precisely the way, the only way in which God is with us and helps us. Matthew

Is There a God in Health Care?
© 2006 by The Haworth Press, Inc. All rights reserved.
doi:10.1300/5554_04

> 8:17 makes it quite clear that Christ helps us, not by virtue of his
> omnipotence, but by virtue of his weakness and suffering.[1]

The "good" that Jesus accomplished, according to the Gospels, brought health to the sick, comfort to the brokenhearted, restoration to life of a young maiden and a widow's son—both dead before their time, peace to the emotionally troubled, and the promise of life after death to those who grieved over their loved ones. Jesus was led by the Holy Spirit of his father, God, to preach of his love for all of creation and of the true nature of faith, namely, compassion for and service of others—giving food, drink, shelter, and comfort in his name—rather than endless recitation of rote prayers or measurable attendance at regular synagogue or temple services. Hence he was able to answer John's disciples in the affirmative when they were sent to ask Jesus if he was the one who was to come or should they look for another. Was he, in other words, the God-sent hope of their nation? Jesus' reply ignores the adulation of the crowds eager for a kingly leader that could have been his. Instead he tells of his compassion for the poor and suffering of the world, his desire to comfort the broken-hearted, to heal the souls of sinners. The wonders worked by him attested not only his Father's special love but also the essence of his own mission on earth which was not at all what the people of his time were expecting. "The blind receive their sight," he told the followers of John the Baptist, "the lame walk, the lepers are cleansed, the deaf hear, the dead are raised, and the poor have good news brought to them" (Matthew 11:5).

This clear application of an earlier prophecy by the revered Isaiah to his own mission was another sign to Jesus' followers that they had to pay attention to the underprivileged, lower-class outcasts of society. Jesus' attitude toward these unfortunates was to be his most alluring and puzzling trait, even as it became a sign of contradiction and disappointment to the more sophisticated hierarchs in Jerusalem or the rebellious zealots who, from their strongholds in the hills of Galilee, were hell-bent to purge the nation of impure pagans. Jesus' predilection for the poor, the sick, and suffering was a way of telling the world of his time that it had waited for the wrong Messiah. Not a sword-wielding, slogan-mouthing, nationalistic liberator, but one who, after having successfully resisted the temptations of power, ambition, and doubt, could urge people to repent of their selfishness and to devote their energies wholly to his Father.

God as caring and near at hand was the center of Jesus' life and the one whom he had so obviously experienced in prayerful intimacy, not as vindictive and judgmental, but as compassionate and so different from the typical religious stereotypes of those without his vision. This was a God who had now drawn humanly near to them, more humanly near than even Jesus himself could adequately express in his Palestinian lifetime. Jesus demanded of his followers that they modify their whole way of thinking about people and all their previous notions about the nature of faith in the Lord God of Israel. The signs of this change of attitude toward God and one another that he preached were to be the healing of physical and mental wounds and the bringing into a brotherly and sisterly communion those who had been separated from one another.

Jesus' answer to John was a stark statement not only of the nature of Jesus' messianic ministry but also of the social mission to be undertaken by those who might claim to have participated in the religious experience of Jesus to the point of wanting to follow him. When studying the Gospels and the letters of Paul, it is not out of order to suggest that the medical profession at its idealistic best continues the healing ministry of Jesus in ways that prayer and attention to God's presence in the life of the physician can make more explicit. Jesus adds a challenge to his words: "Blessed is anyone who takes no offense at me" (Matthew 11:6). They are indeed blessed who are not ashamed or embarrassed to assume the same difficult mission of Jesus and have the courage to risk everything in this mission. Here those who claim to be Christians, especially those in the healing professions, must ask themselves if what they do in their personal lives and in their practice constitute good news to the disadvantaged and weakest citizens of contemporary society. Against the attitude of relating to people under the paralyzing aegis of law or under the influence of class-conscious stereotypes or in terms of their monetary productivity, the early Christian community proposed the example of Jesus for whom the sinner, the diseased, the outcast, and the poor were the object of his special concern. Unfortunately, these are also the very people many Christians of later centuries, including our own, have been inclined to avoid or write off, pious prayers for them and continued claims to be good Christian churchgoers to the contrary notwithstanding.

CARE OF THE POOR AND THE SICK

Jesus' ministry was filled with wonders, challenges to think differently about people their society despised, and to approach the problems of life with new hope. He was a courageous prophet-leader unabashed in confronting authoritarian arrogance and speaking up for those who had no real voice in society, which enhanced Jesus' attractive, caring personality before the impoverished masses. Matthew, speaking for his mostly Jewish community, tells us that Rabbi Jesus held the crowds spellbound because he spoke with authority, unlike the typical religious leaders of his day. He had a special, heartfelt tenderness toward the sick, knowing that in addition to their physical ills they were also tormented by the inhumane, popular judgment that their sufferings signed God's enmity toward and ultimate disdain of them. This was a troubling judgment, not at all unlike the attitudes toward the destitute on welfare, the "unproductive" elderly, and the leprous AIDS (acquired immunodeficiency syndrome) patients who are still being ostracized today. Jesus detested and denounced the ideological rationalization that the mainstream religion of his day had pronounced on these unfortunates, concluding simplistically that they were being punished by God for their sins. Jesus braved the indignation and supercilious opposition of the temple authorities in order to heal these sick outcasts who sought him out as their only hope to be restored to wholeness and respectability.

In the Gospel portrait of Jesus, his communion with God led him not just into the deserts and onto the mountaintops to pray but into the villages to treat people with the same compassionate concern that he claimed was the true, loving nature of his Father. The people of whatever class he met were his brothers and sisters in ways as deep as the mysterious irresistible spirit of God's love. Jesus' days and dreams were filled with that intense personal outreach of concern for the hurting among his people that always seemed to leave him restless. He was a man driven by such a hunger and thirst for justice that he was considered mad by his friends and relatives (see Mark 3:20). The stories he told seemed to flow naturally and powerfully from his prayerful intimacy with his Father that was the taproot of his own sense of being. At times this burst into such uncommon expression, not certified by the religious leadership, that many called him a blasphemer. If not "blasphemy," then his words were at least outrageous.

The God of the coming Kingdom, Jesus declared, is a God of unbelievable tenderness, forbearance, and forgiveness—all essential qualities of the healing professions! His was a God quite novel to the people of Jesus' day as also to those of today who clamor for judicial vengeance and unmerciful executions of criminals. Jesus' God was the brokenhearted Father who waited at the road for the return of his prodigal son, the softhearted dad who does not even allow the renegade son to get the words out asking for forgiveness but clasps him in a tearful embrace and covers him with kisses. Most Christians today would share more in the indignation of the older son than in Jesus' admiration for a Father who lacks a "proper" sense of justice and willingness to punish.

But, then, Jesus adds to his description the baffling note that his Father is excessive in generosity and quite willing to disregard principles of strict justice in order to grant the latecomer on the job everything he has given to those who have labored all day long (Matthew 20:1-16). Jesus' Father will enrich even those who seem most undeserving of such generosity. If this is offensive to one's sense of getting ahead in the business world, then Jesus can follow with a portrayal of the "Shepherd God" recklessly abandoning ninety-nine sheep to go looking for the one lost (Luke 15:4-7). This could hardly be considered prudent by any audience of sheepherders, yet it is a mind-captivating metaphor of the way his Father simply cannot give up on any of the children who might have strayed away from a Father's providential care.

One can only wonder how Jesus' story would go over with health care providers when medical coverage and medicine are limited to those only who can afford it or whose systems of triage would certainly leave that one lost sheep (symbolic of the ostracized and those considered socially wayward) to fend for itself. The high cost of medicine sometimes impinges on a person's food, at times forcing the choice: supper or medicine?

HEALTH CARE PROVIDERS

Doctors and others involved in the healing professions can be viewed, in their compassionate outreach to the hurting of today's societies, as following Jesus in caring for people overburdened with physical, mental, and spiritual ills. Jesus' challenge—"greater things shall you do"—applies in a particular way to those who are entrusted with easing the pain and sufferings of those who have become their "patients." Those in the healing professions, similar to Jesus, are themselves asked to do the unexpected in a "me first" society, to allow themselves to be inconvenienced, even troubled, by those whom God has placed in their care, and to make time for demanding people when they themselves might be craving nothing more than rest and quiet. Older clinicians have pointed out that the most important thing for someone starting medical practice is being available.

In a remarkable passage from his spiritual classic *Life Together,* Dietrich Bonhoeffer described this availability to be for the other as part of the essence of belonging to a Christian community. He calls this the great service of "active helpfulness" which holds a community together.

> Nobody is too good for the lowest service. Those who worry about the loss of time entailed by such small, external acts of helpfulness are usually taking their own work too seriously. We must be ready to allow ourselves to be interrupted by God, who will thwart our plans and frustrate our ways time and again, even daily, by sending people across our path with their demands and requests. We can, then, pass them by, preoccupied with our more important daily tasks, just as the priest—perhaps reading the Bible—passed by the man who had fallen among robbers. When we do that, we pass by the visible sign of the cross raised in our lives to show us that God's way, and not our own, is what counts.[2]

This passage was meant originally for seminarians about to enter into a subversive church ministry in the midst of their enemies in Nazi Germany, and called upon to rescue Jews from their fate in the death camps. His text speaks also of the sacrifices demanded of those who would work in the healing professions in the prayerful way that has been suggested by Doctor Bill. During his imprisonment prior to his execution, Bonhoeffer called Jesus, the "man for others," and proclaimed that the church was the church only when it lived, as did Jesus, to be of service to others. Could this not be an apt description of those engaged in the healing professions?

THE PROBLEMS OF SUFFERING AND DEATH

The story of Jesus offers a unique depiction of the problems of suffering and death that every healer has to deal with. As instructed in the Gospels, Jesus, the prophetic healer and "wonder worker," later to be hailed by Christians as their savior, was not immune himself from the human condition that harbored the seeds of its own vulnerability, weakness, deterioration, and death. Jesus suffered. Mark's description of Jesus' agony is bracing in its starkness. Jesus, he wrote, was desperately depressed at his impending fate. In Mark's words, "Horror and dismay came over him, and he said to them, 'my heart is ready to break with grief'" (Mark 14:33-35, NEB).[3] This was surely a prophet from God who had fully embraced human weakness.

We must keep the Gospel account of the death of Jesus in mind when we deal with the reality of death. Jesus' sufferings took him to the brink of despair when, experiencing the painful loneliness of the prophet surrounded by hatred and seemingly abandoned to a dreadful fate, he cried from the cross: "My God, my God, why have you forsaken me?" (Matthew 27:46). Yet Jesus died with that prayer of trust on his lips: "Father, into your hands I commend my spirit" (Luke 23:46), which summed up his whole life of faith. He died continuing to love and trust his Father, confident that his death was the hidden accomplishment of his mission, as the martyrdom of the prophets and the sufferings of the Just One's of Israel eventually vindicated their message and their lives became an example to future generations.

After the experience of Jesus' being raised from the dead to become, as Paul declared, "a life-giving spirit," his followers believed Jesus was still present, sharing meals with them once again. Their lives were transformed by his resurrection. Jesus' words at their farewell meal the night before his execution, once so distressing in his announcement that he was leaving them, came back to them with electrifying impact. "It is to your advantage that I go away, for if I do not go away, the Advocate will not come to you; but if I go away, I will send him to you" (John 16:7). Puzzling, disturbing words, indeed! It was better, Jesus informed them, that he disappear from sight as he did physically. Is there any Christian who might not wish for Jesus to be always accessible in some central location, perhaps similar to the pope in Rome? Imagine the salivating of travel agents hawking pilgrimages, the steady flow of the wounded, physically and emotionally, to the greatest healer of them all, or the soul-salving gifts from the wealthy parcel posted to Jesus Savior! If a Texas millionaire could give an oil well to two of Britain's richest members of the royal family on their wedding days, think of the gifts that would be heaped on Rabbi Jesus, savior, miracle worker, hailed by Christians as judge of all the world and its pretensions! If readers like the idea of a single Pope Rabbi Jesus for all time, they have missed the whole point of Jesus' declaration why it was better for him to be physically off the scene.

HEALING AS CHRIST DOES

Jesus insists that he must join God in physical invisibility so that their spirit of love and truth, their healing power, can transform people into being Christ for every succeeding generation. The "truth" of the Holy Spirit is that Jesus does not leave his followers. He enters into communion with every believer while his spirit begins in them the ages-long process of their reaching out to all peoples searching for and caring for the Jesus Christ incognito in the foreign lands, slums, prisons, and killing fields, to name only part of their mission. Jesus' followers are called to affirm the Christ in the destitute, the people of color, the convict on a death row in Texas, the Jews in Nazi death camps, the lepers of Molokai, the dying, disease-ridden poor of Calcutta, to name only a handful of those with whom Jesus identifies as the least of his brothers and sisters and with whom he has made common cause. When they met to break the bread and drink the cup of the Lord's supper, they reminded themselves through this simple ritual that Jesus was still in their midst. They were empowered to see Jesus in one another. And their mission was to seek out the Christ in the lost children and the unfortunate multitudes who had never been exposed to the beauty of Jesus of Nazareth and to the healing power of Jesus' spirit.

The faith of Jesus can be comforting to those believers who must bear the burden of seeing a loved one suffer and die or, in the case of a medical caregiver, watching the steady deterioration that will inevitably end in the death of a beloved patient. God's answer to the so-called "problem of suffering" is not a well-refined theology or a "can't fail" prayer for deliverance. God does not offer any glib, divinely guaranteed explanations for the tormenting moments when human grief can only weep in helplessness. God chooses to suffer with those who suffer. Jesus did not ask his Father to send the twelve legions of angels to make body parts of the arresting temple guards; nor did he call down fire and brimstone on the Roman soldiers mocking him in his humiliating, pain-filled agony.

Physicians and caregivers, too, may suffer with those whom they are trying to comfort, as we have pointed out in our description of why doctors should no longer refrain from drawing close to their patients in their illness. Indeed, by praying with their patients, doctors can help God become a consoling presence for them in their sufferings. The thought that God, too, bears the hurts and rejections of the innocent, that God suffers with all his children, and is a hidden presence even in their lonely, degraded deaths at the hands of a criminal ideology, inspired in many Christian martyrs that extraordinary peace of mind that even their executioners could only wonder at.

The man of sorrows rejected to die on the cross is the image of God's own sorrowing in the evil choices of God's children. The cross of Christ symbolizes God's own involvement in the problem of human suffering. In effect, God offers no simple answer to this problem; he suffers with us and promises resurrection of the just.

THE INEVITABILITY OF THE CROSS: GEFF'S EXPERIENCE

Despite the consolation offered in the story of Jesus' death-resurrection experience, the more frightening reality is that there is for Jesus, as for us, no resurrection without the cross. Daniel Sulmasy points out that

> health care professionals can make the Way of the Cross every day. They see patients live out their own unique passion plays, subsumed under the passion of Christ. . . . They see patients unjustly condemned to painful diagnoses. . . . They see them take up huge crosses that they do not deserve. They see the women, always the women, who attend to the most basic needs of the

dying in their final hours and days. They hear the dying cry out in prayers of warning for all the living . . .[4]

Sulmasy goes on to say that these same physicians "can see Christ in every patient's Golgotha . . . if they can see the resurrection that is promised for all who suffer in love, they know that God is with them in their work."[5] Sulmasy also offers a valuable spiritual insight to health caregivers when they become confused at the suffering of their patients or given over to fear and insecurity or even disillusionment with the practice of medicine. They can learn from their patients that God is present in them, reaching out to the physician, nurses, others involved in their treatments for the care that the least of Jesus' brothers and sisters crave at that moment.

Theologians can also learn about the presence of God and the way God in Jesus Christ has identified with what we may consider the least of Jesus' brothers and sisters. It sometimes takes the woundedness of the would-be healer to open the heart to this unbelievably touching mode of God's being with God's children in those crisis moments when the human body is at its weakest or in passage from this life to life eternal. One such experience has led me to claim that I learned more about God's love for us through little children terminally ill from cancers of all sorts than I ever did from any of the many heady or pious analyses of suffering and death in the learned tomes of theology that I had studied and mastered. I knew the words that could explain the difference between the ultimate and the here-and-now, between the misery of today and eternal happiness, between the momentary pain and the joy of life everlasting.

As we were ready to welcome our third child into our family, our own way of the cross began. Our lovely daughter, Susan, then three and a half years old, had been ill off and on with mysterious ailments that included frequent falling, clumsiness to the point of dragging her left foot, headaches, early morning vomiting, and noticeable lethargy. We were hoping for something we could deal with, perhaps through exercise and physical fitness. But when the early morning vomiting became more frequent and accompanied by severe headaches we demanded to see a specialist. We were referred to a neurologist who immediately ordered a CT scan as early as possible the next day.

Susan was drugged so she would be immobile for the brain scan; Joan was home with baby Michael; I was going through heartbreak in the waiting room. I had taken this trusting child who had no idea of the ordeals she was about to endure, hiding from her the overpowering fear of the worst possible diagnosis. As soon as the neurologist called me out of the waiting room, I sensed that something was wrong. The doctor informed me that Susan was suffering from a massive brain tumor rising out of her brainstem and that she needed emergency surgery. She would not leave the hospital for another three weeks. Joan was driven to the hospital; baby Michael was left in the care of Joan's sister. My sister-in-law took Brendan, our middle child, to her home in Orange, New Jersey. Her three children showered him with affection and fun.

Receiving the news was traumatic enough. Holding our daughter as the nurses took her blood, jabbing her with needles for the first time in her life, was the saddest thing we had ever had to do with her. No amount of my hugging and speaking soothing words of reassurance could allay her fears and pain. She became a frightened child in a hostile environment, hurt by people who were trying only to help her, and her mommy and daddy unable to protect her. At times, too, we had to leave her with nurses while we conferred with the neurologist, the neurosurgeon, the anesthesiologist team, and the interns on her ward in preparation for the emergency surgery she was to undergo the next day. We were told that without the surgery she would die. The surgery lasted nine-and-a-half hours. The highly skilled neurosurgeon could remove only enough of it to ease the pressure on her brain. The tumor had already penetrated the brainstem, so the rest had to be fought for the next two years through chemotherapy.

After only two weeks of chemotherapy with her resistance level reduced to zero, she contracted meningitis. Her brain had swollen so much we were told she would probably not live through night. It had been my turn to sleep on the cot by her bedside so she would know that her daddy or mommy were nearby. Joan was summoned to the hospital, not knowing if she would find Susan alive or dead. Susan was rescued when a quick-thinking neurosurgeon on call ran into the treatment room and plunged a syringe into her head and removed several vials of cerebral fluid. I stood by in total shock. There followed an emergency surgery to install a permanent shunt—permanent only in the sense she would always need a shunt. In the years that followed she would have to submit to nine more surgeries to replace nonfunctioning shunts, each surgery requiring her to learn to walk unaided all over again after a time in either a wheelchair or using a walker.

I spent much of that year in the hospital with her. It often fell to me to be with Susan to hold and hug her while the needles were inserted and the toxic chemicals released into her frail body. She was not the only child I held; some mothers could not bring themselves to watch while their children, usually crying pitifully, would be administered the chemotherapy. My heart was broken many times over, although I struggled to control my emotions lest my own upset be picked up by the children. I did not mind the effort of comforting these sick children, but I resented the pain these beautiful children were suffering and my having to witness the steady deterioration of those destined to die young. I read aloud to them in the huge waiting room decorated with Disney characters and equipped with a large birdcage and fish tank, things to distract the youngsters from the painful treatments that awaited them. Most of the sad moments of those years have been buried in my subconscious, to surface during occasional nightmares and at times when they intrude into my meditations. Some incidents have remained vivid in my memory.

My anxious prayers that the chemotherapy would be so effective she would be completely healed, were not answered the way I wanted. Her life on four different occasions would remain on a precarious edge when we were told her chances of survival were dim. As a former religious with vows of poverty, chastity, and obedience, for twenty years of my life I had been trained in the art of prayer. As a spiritual director I taught young postulants and novices how to pray. But there in the hospital waiting out the long hours of surgery and the periods of chemotherapy, I was unable to pray with any conviction. I had stopped saying the Rosary years before, but upon putting my hand in my coat pocket for some inexplicable reason I felt a small pouch containing my old rosary. I began to pray the Rosary, something I could do without thinking. The simple words of the Our Father and the Hail Mary, known by rote, became my main distraction. This helped me as I fretted the hours away. Prayer helped me during the hours when I was on the horrific treadmill of holding Susan while nurses took her blood and plunged the stinging chemicals into her bloodstream, when her tears mingled with mine. When my prayers for Susan's recovery went unanswered, the struggle within me took the turn of my being angry at God who permitted such a thing to happen to Susan and these innocent children.

A RELIGIOUS EXPERIENCE

All was not a continual bleakness. There were moments when Susan seemed to perk up and when the doctors announced they were pleased with her progress. We made friends with other families who were with us in a kind of fellowship of suffering. We were closest to the family of little Charlie, who had been in the same ward as Susan. Charlie had been diagnosed with ocular cancer that with every seeming successful treatment transmuted into a cancer in some other part of his body. Charlie and Susan became fast friends, like brother and sister; they even bickered like siblings. I liked to read to Charlie and Frankie, another boy, freckle-faced and full of fun, who died later that year of lung cancer. As Susan seemed to grow stronger, Charlie, who arrived at the hospital invariably wearing a superman shirt, grew weaker and his sufferings became more intense. Finally, one day at the end of winter, his doctor told me she was going to inform the parents that they were going to stop his chemotherapeutic treatments. Given his weakened state, the chemicals were only making him weaker and intensifying his sufferings; Charlie was terminal. The physicians had decided to tell the parents this, knowing Charlie would be surrounded with love and care until the end. I understood the compassion behind this step; Charlie had suffered. But what was happening only intensified my anger with God.

And so very naturally when Charlie's parents were asked to confer with the doctor I took Charlie by the hand so he could sit on my lap and I could read to him. But Charlie wanted no part of this. He cried, begging for his Mom and Dad. He made so much noise that I took him into a side room. Susan came with me, dressed as was our wont in a miniature doctor's uniform—one of the doctors used to take Susan with her on her rounds with the other children to put them at ease and to make Susan feel important. Charlie's crying became louder and anything I tried only made him more desperate to be with his parents. Susan patted him and told him not to cry, that his mommy and daddy were coming back soon. As for me, my anger, sadness, and frustration was near fission as nothing I tried succeeded in consoling Charlie.

Then, all of a sudden, it happened. I went into a kind of trance, as if I had fainted. A strange light seemed to fill the room. I saw my whole life flit before me from the little steps that had changed my life into its many directions, to the loneliness that convinced me to leave religious life. Every moment seemed to be connected, all fitting into one pattern guided by some power beyond my control. My life came back to me as a whole with everything strangely connected and an irresistible, loving force keeping it and me all together. It was a wholeness I had never experienced before. Then a voice came at me or within me—I do not know—but it was a voice that pierced the kaleidoscopic events streaming into my consciousness with suddenness and power. The voice said, "If it were not for me you would not be here in this place holding this child of mine." Then just as it came upon me the light went away, the events of my life ceased to pass before me, and I came out of it. And when I came to, Charlie was asleep in my arms and Susan was looking at me as if I had fallen asleep too. Charlie's parents came back to take him home. He died peacefully two months later.

At his funeral service, I took Susan to see Charlie one more time. This time he was lying in a coffin, dressed in the Superman outfit that he loved to wear. She said out loud something that provoked many sobs among the congregation: "Oh look, there's Charlie. I'm going to kiss him and make him all better." Susan was only four years old.

I have tried again and again to recapture that moment of my intense religious experience. I have asked the Lord in prayer to give it back to me just one more time so I can experience again the peace of soul and sense of being guided by the loving care of the Holy Spirit who reminded me so forcefully that God does indeed care for the little children who suffer from the same illnesses as adults and some of whom will die young. God works gently through all the decisions we make, all the turns our lives take, even our own sins, to lead us to where God will have us be at a given moment. What appears to be an accidental occurrence or some wanton act of chance or luck is still enshrouded in the providential presence of God. That experience convinced me that God never ceases to look out for his children, providing at given moments those who will be the arms, the laps, the hugs, the compassion that God continues through those who, similar to Jesus, become the incarnation of the divine presence in the lives of those who beg God for deliverance from their pain. God condescended to my own weakness and reminded me that my anger was misdirected and that I did not understand at all the sufferings that God endures in order that we might be free even from the possibility of the divine tampering with nature, that even death will not have the last word in this life so destined to be transcended into life eternal.

DOCTOR BILL'S EXPERIENCES

My first class with Geff as a graduate student at La Salle University, "The Teaching Healing Ministry of Jesus," was a shocker in that he announced that his daughter, Susan, was suffering from a brain tumor. He informed us that this might cause him to miss a class before the end of the semester. During one of our classes he poured out from his heart the cross he was carrying concerning Susan. My first thought was that here was a man, whom God had allowed to be "broken," and now he has become vulnerable and "open" to so many others, including us students. These are qualities that need to be found among the followers of Jesus no matter what ancillary vocation they choose. As individuals we can be too "zipped up," which can cause us to block out deeper levels of compassion and empathy for those who are hurting. In my case it can make health caregivers awkward in accepting love from our patients and friends or less than open in expressing our own love. The good thing about being broken, as I have mentioned earlier, is that, once an individual suffers any sort of unexpected loss, a transformation often follows, a depth of caring not present before, a push along the spiritual journey. Suffering can make us more compassionate of others and help us attain the enhanced sense of wholeness that caregivers need.

But this does not obviate the question of why God allows good people to suffer in the first place. Here we encounter both God's mystery and, at the same time, God's promise to accompany, console, and bring healing to the afflicted. This may not be the answer we prefer, but we accept it on faith. Often a serious and unexpected loss, be it loss of good health, spouse, job, finances, integrity, or being suddenly unable to handle a tragedy, such as the tragedy of the collapse of the Twin Towers on September 11, 2001, or before any number of severe unexpected losses will likely bring about the death to what was previously our all important "self." This can result in a sudden return to or renewed reliance on an all-loving God.

CARRYING THE CROSS: WE ARE NOT ALONE

One of the most difficult tasks for a caregiver is looking after a family member who lives with chronic illness or handicap. We all may experience carrying the cross for another, but we can consider ourselves blessed if the interval is not too long or harsh. At times God appears to reward this experience by enhancing our spiritual growth as a caregiver. Some of these difficult medical conditions would certainly include the caretaker spouse who devotes a good part of the day's routine to caring for the partner handicapped by Alzheimer's disease. For many others it is the constant care one must devote to those who suffer from incapacitating Parkinson's disease, patients requiring frequent dialysis for renal failure, the refractory heart patient who is not a candidate for a heart transplant, the hepatitis C patient who has developed cirrhosis of the liver (as was the case with my father), stroke patients with severe residual speech and paralysis, or the child born with a severe handicap.

John Nash's long struggle with mental illness, portrayed in the movie *A Beautiful Mind,* illustrates in one small way how one person can be God's help to another. Nash was able to overcome severe schizophrenia, but in the process, there was the equally dramatic assistance that required endurance, love, and courage on the part of his wife. The film revealed her patience and perseverance as well as her frustrations throughout the saga until Nash regained his mind and became well enough to receive the Nobel Prize for Economics. This was a deeply touching film and there was not a dry eye among many of us at its conclusion.[6] The quiet heroism found in the hearts of so many caregivers and patients alike in dealing with long-term illnesses has always impressed me as a standing testimonial to their fortitude and God's grace inspiring them to be God's own compassionate outreach to his hurting children.

Many patients cared for by a practicing physician are trying to survive and prevail following a severe stroke, accident, or any kind of illness that leaves the imprint of a serious disability. How people react to this "cross" with an uncommon courage and even sense of humor is always heartwarming to health care providers, leading many of us to acknowledge that we often receive greater gifts from our patients than we could ever give them. This, I believe, is God's way of making the difficulties encountered in health care bearable and even rewarding to the caregivers.

One of my patients, a sixty-year-old carpenter, whom I will call Jerry, and who had been diagnosed with a progressive neurological disorder at the age of fifty, soon came to grips with the progressive difficulty he experienced in walking as well as enunciating words. This resulted in his early retirement with disability. Nevertheless, he continued to volunteer five days a week in a local hospital. During each visit Jerry would always say to the patients, "I am a volunteer; I am also a good listener. I'd be happy to make a phone call or run an errand to the hospital gift shop for anything you might need." This helpful outreach to others prevented his centering upon his own diagnosis. I watched Jerry travel the road of his remaining years as his disability progressed from the initial unsteady gait, to the reliance upon a cane, and ultimately to a wheelchair existence. He was both admired and a source of inspiration for everyone he met and spoke to. Helping others gave him a sense of purpose as well as pleasure. I am sure the inner peace he gained greatly slowed down the disease's progression that went on for twenty-five years. Untold similar cases could be told of patients with a host of different illnesses who carry on and even blossom under the stress of an unfavorable diagnosis with little hope for a pain free future.

Michael J. Fox is another such person. His book *Lucky Man: A Memoir* describes his continuing to remain active in theater and movies despite the physical handicap of Parkinson's disease.[7] As a guest on *Larry King Live,* Fox reiterated that his disease was a "gift," as he tries to live each day more fully and to appreciate his life and career much more. He now devotes much time and talent toward continued research in this field. Fox, by accepting his disease and moving forward in spite of it, has shared his "gift" with countless others and given hope to untold people who are themselves coping with the ravaging effects of Parkinson's disease. Fox and Jerry are but two examples of the many who have been blessed with the urge to go forward and contribute, each in their unique way, to the good of society regardless of the uncertain future they have faced and embraced as a "gift."

DO NOT BLAME GOD FOR OUR ILLS

The acute loss of life, as in accidents, with no time for good-byes has always raised the question: Why did God let this happen? The question can eat at the hearts of family members and friends for months and years. Some leave their churches and synagogues. Our faith reminds us that God remains mysterious in so many of life's vicissitudes. God creates the earth and its creatures and gives us the freedom to make our own decisions in nearly every area of life. God is not responsible for evil acts by evil people or accidents that are in line with the laws of nature. These can be seen as by-products of our free choices for good and ill. The Bible reminds us that God allows the rain to fall on the good and the evil alike for we are all God's children and are loved despite our many failings (see Matthew 5:45).

From another point of view, tragic, even premature deaths often do lead to contributions to the common good. For example, donor organs obtained from suitable individuals who have recently died can give a "second life" to very ill and incapacitated individuals waiting for a specific organ, perhaps a heart, kidney, liver, lung, or bone marrow. A living person, for example, can donate the right lobe of his or her liver to a patient suffering from liver failure. The liver has the ability to regenerate on its own in the donor as well as the recipient. With the advent of genetic engineering, stem cells from the bone marrow can be directed to repair some damaged organs. New coronary arteries may one day replace the damaged ones located in the heart. This is a whole new field that is being clinically developed even as I write these words.

A given tragedy can bring about a transition away from our innate selfishness with all of its power, prestige, and material wealth as the true goal of success, and help us arrive at a point of leaning more upon God and God's word for a sense of meaning in our lives. This can be a difficult and unfamiliar road to travel. Yet, God's gracious presence can help us attain the inner peace that might have eluded us for most of our lives, the gift that no amount of money can purchase. Many times, following prayers for healing among patients admitted with heart problems, for example, there occurs a "letting go," a surrender to God during which healing is expedited and inner peace attained. This is a common experience in the CCU, when we are dealing with a patient just admitted following a heart attack, if we are able to discern that the patient is open to an audible prayer for healing. From personal experience and by examining the monitor at the head of the bed, we can visualize the anxiety causing an adrenalin rush that can be damaging to the heart because of increased pulse rate and elevated blood pressure and heart palpitations. Following prayer, the patient often sighs as a manifestation of his or her "letting go" and letting God take over. This is accompanied by a drop in the pulse rate and greatly improved cardiac rhythm. Can this principle be expanded to more people, not just those who are critically ill?

Human suffering appears to be inevitable in all of our lives. Our professions as physician and teacher attest that suffering is a worldwide reality of human existence. A clergyperson from a Christian church in Manhattan once quoted in his sermon a question published by *The London Times* in 1910. The question was directed to a number of authors and essayists of that era and read: "What is wrong with the world?" Gilbert Keith Chesterton, one of the writers and celebrated author of religious tracts, had the shortest response: "Dear sirs: I am. Sincerely yours, G. K. Chesterton."[8] A good question to pose to ourselves about what is wrong with our world: "Are we?"

What can one do, faced with the seeming all pervasiveness of suffering in our world? Some examples come to mind. Months after America's own descent into a "valley of death's darkness," the Reverend Lyndon Harris wrote an inspiring account of God's sparing Trinity Church's St. Paul's Chapel from destruction. The chapel became a shelter for an outpouring of care and love by thousands of people from all over the United States and other parts of the world after the events of September 11. The media referred to St. Paul's Chapel, located directly across from the World Trade Center, as "The Miracle of St. Paul's."[9] The chapel, although covered with dust and debris, survived without sustaining even a crack in the stained glass windows. The doors remained open twenty-four hours daily serving the host of volunteers, firefighters, police, medical personnel, as well as a multitude of caregivers such as grief counselors, podiatrists, massage therapists, clergy, food handlers, and the military. Two thousand meals were served there each day. By Easter 2002, 400,000 free meals had been given out, involving 5,000 volunteers. Part of the success has been both financial and hands-on help from many institutions, relief organizations, from individuals in this country, and resources from all over the globe.

Another "miracle" that occurred at the World Trade Center that received worldwide coverage seemed to take place in the appearance of a perfectly formed cross created by two damaged and interconnected steel beams, standing tall above all the wreckage and smoke. When I visited the area in March of 2002, the presence of that cross seemed to be more magnified and towering as the underlying debris was continually being removed. It struck me as a Christian that here was a sign of hope from God amid the chaos of buildings in ruins and lives destroyed. Here, too, was a symbol of the nonviolent, forgiving Christ who enjoined on his followers to be peacemakers in this troubled world. A year later it was difficult to see this nation hastening, not to understand the causes of the hatred of those who perpetrated the senseless slaughter of American citizens, but to kill those responsible through a campaign of bombing and a resort to war that would, in turn, take thousands of lives. We might ask if we, in the aftermath of September 11, learned the lessons of our own vulnerability and the need to be compassionate toward others, even our enemies?

The Pew Research Center study of the event revealed that, with the memory of September 11 ever present in our minds, and with the fear of more terrorist attacks hanging over our heads, many people turned again to religion, trusting in God's grace for the necessary strength and courage to cope with adversity and to seek in God alone the ultimate power beyond our human resources. Other studies have concluded that seven out of ten Americans are praying more, and places of worship have noted a significant increase in attendance. Often a spurt in church attendance can be correlated with a jump in the level of anxiety from impending danger or news of terror attacks killing Americans on a global scale. A related question would be whether the increased church attendance has also been accompanied by more acts of charity, compassion, volunteering, and genuine love for one another.

The story of Lisa Beamer, now a widow with two small children, is a strong testimony to our need for God in times of tragedy. Her husband, Todd, was a leader of the passengers who struggled with the terrorists on Flight 93 as it headed in the direction of the capital on September 11. His voice captured the imagination of the country with the words, "Let's roll," as he and others fought the men who had taken over control of the plane. All were killed as the plane plunged into a field in western Pennsylvania. Speaking to a Christian forum at Princeton University, Lisa mentioned that it was her Christian faith, instilled in her as a young child, that enabled her to bear the deep anguish that overwhelmed her following her young husband's tragic death. Today her husband's last words, "Let's roll," have become memorialized as an exhortation to combat evil. Concluding her talk, she urged those in the audience to open their hearts to God in order to live a richer and comforting life.[10]

The importance of starting our young children in a loving attitude of faith which can serve as an anchor later in the many storms and uncertainties of life has been shown time and again to be of prime importance in parenting. We must treasure those individuals that touch the hearts of children and teach the early lessons of fair play and compassion, thereby allowing them to have the best opportunity to develop into caring adults and to contribute their unique gifts toward creating the better society we often dream about.

The late Fred Rogers was able to touch the hearts of impressionable children in a way that dovetailed with the tasks of parenting that Lisa now faces without the presence of her heroic husband. Mr. Rogers told stories, wrote songs, and in his low-key voice passed on simple lessons of love, wisdom, compassion, and even some of life's problems in a way that children could readily understand. During his lifetime he became the recipient of innumerable awards for his work. Mr. Rogers died of stomach cancer, February 27, 2003, at age seventy-four. As a young boy, he was a very shy child, apparently lacking self-confidence, never taking the center stage in school activities. Yet he had a special relationship with his grandfather, whom he frequently visited. His grandfather made it a point to praise Fred, to enhance his self-confidence and sense of self-worth. Mr. Rogers remembered the positive influence his grandfather had made upon him, both as a child and during his adulthood, when working with children. He often referred to a certain letter he received from his grandfather that pointed out the great joy he experienced whenever Rogers visited him. He also remarked that he did not want his grandson, Fred, to change in any way. He emphasized that he was loved—"just the way you are." Rogers learned how important it was for young children to experience being loved and affirmed; it was the best way for a child to build self-confidence.[11] It seems to me that, as adults and caregivers, it would also be well for us to let others know how much we appreciate them despite their

various degrees of illness and reactions to our well-intentioned ministrations.

In these reflections, we have attempted to discover a constant amid
the tragic turns our lives can take. Not everyone is blessed with a reassuring religious experience or the kind of faith that remains strong
when health crises, terminal illness, or even victimization through violence create enough chaos to rob us of our serenity and plunge us
into a spiral of sadness and near despair. The stories of Jesus, the biblical account of God's providential care despite the evil that still
haunts this world, the compassionate outreach of people of faith, and
the personal strength that God bestows in times of illness and the loss
of a loved one all attest to the continued presence and steadfast love of
God despite all appearances to the contrary. The faith that is the central dynamic in the healing process remains God's great gift in life's
search for meaning.

DISCUSSION QUESTIONS

1. Can we share brief stories of what Jesus Christ means to us from
   our reading of the Gospels?
2. Why did Jesus Christ refuse to be a kingly leader in order to become more a healer of the poor and needy?
3. Describe Jesus' Father. How was this God different from the typical religious stereotypes extent in Jesus' time? Today?
4. Why was Jesus able to hold the crowds spellbound when preaching in his own day? Would this be true today in the issues of social justice, peace, and war?
5. Explain how and why Jesus' personal qualities are also essential
   qualities in the healing and health care professions.
6. How and why can the stories of Jesus' suffering and death help
   health care and hospice care workers in their ministries?
7. Comment on how God does care for the terminally ill through a
   wide variety of healings.
8. Comment on why God allows good people to suffer. Use examples of the death of children, the tragedy of September 11, and
   other stories of God drawing good out of evil.
9. Why should we not blame God for our illnesses and sufferings?

10. Why is it important to instill in the young the early lessons of fair play, compassion, and caring for others? Are prisons filled with those whose childhood was bereft of such care? Compare the costs of incarcerating criminals with the cost of educating children properly in their formative years. How does this connect with Jesus Christ's compassion for the outcasts of society?

Chapter 5

Suffering, Terminal Illness, and the Healing Ministry

No reassuring literature can ever remove fully the fright and frustration of coping with chronic suffering and terminal illness. The personal testimonies of those who have been in the dark valley of progressive physical deterioration can only offer at best examples of the courage that might ease somewhat the fear of the unknown in those whose physical and emotional strength is slowly ebbing away. Tending to the needs of those who are suffering from chronic or terminal illness is a major concern for all health caregivers. This is a primary goal in all stages of medical illness, whether it is an acute condition, a chronic one, or a terminal case. In addition to the obvious ministrations of the family doctor, a wide variety of vocations are involved today in dealing with the suffering patient. The ministry of health care has, in fact, become interdisciplinary, a cooperative effort involving medicine, law, ethics, counseling, religion, public health, social work, public policy, hospital administration, pharmacology, and physiotherapy. In today's medical systems, the primary care physician is usually the director of this coalition.

SUFFERING IN THE CONTEXT OF THE PURPOSE OF ONE'S LIFE

Unfortunately, it often takes a shock such as an unexpected, debilitating illness or personal loss to free us sufficiently to reevaluate our lives and to answer the question: "What is the purpose of my life?" or from a theological point of view, "What might God be trying to tell me?" God does have a plan for each of us, but so often we are too busy

Is There a God in Health Care?
© 2006 by The Haworth Press, Inc. All rights reserved.
doi:10.1300/5554_05

93

with our secular concerns to hear God's word. Notwithstanding our deafness at times to God's call to us, faith never ceases to assure us that God cares for us as beloved children whether we are well, suffering from physical or emotional disabilities, or even terminally ill.

The problem of suffering yields no easy answers. Not even in the death of Jesus was there at the time any clear-cut rationale to explain just why he had to suffer. Was it really God's will rather than the suffering inflicted by an evil, imperial system on the innocent Jesus? Indeed, God does not offer any compelling answer to the problem of suffering or evil. Instead, a more contemporary theology declares that God suffers with us. In the biblical word, God has, in fact, claimed to be victimized in the persecution of God's innocent children. God enters into communion with those who suffer and die at the climax of their journey back to him. This is an individual journey as well as a communal journey because of our connectedness in faith with God's ways for us. We can be helped in understanding the why of it all by the stories of those who have traveled those last stages of their life's journey toward life everlasting and, in their own afflictions, they have at least served to remove part of the mystery of how people react to and cope with suffering and terminal illness.

One such person is Philip Simmons, who, at thirty-five years old, was diagnosed with ALS (amyotrophic lateral sclerosis) better known as Lou Gehrig's disease. Knowing that his prognosis was guarded, Simmons's book, *Learning to Fall,* concerns itself more about living in the moment rather than dwelling about his neurological condition. He arrived at a stage where he could accept his condition. This condition, among other symptoms, causes a progressive loss of balance, and frequent falls, hence the appropriateness of the book's title. The heart of the book relates to the process of taking leave of his earthly attachments. In the process he rediscovered a profound freedom. This enabled him to live more freely in the present, to better appreciate and cope with the vicissitudes of everyday life.[1]

The example of how Simmons found meaning and peace in handling his own incurable disease does not eliminate the perennial question of such suffering. Is there a higher purpose in all this? Some have suggested that their illness has become their "wake-up call" to examine more deeply their purpose in life or the possibility that God may be calling them to enter into a new direction in their service of others. Some of those involved in Alcoholics Anonymous (AA) have witnessed individuals being lifted out of their own vomit while lying in a stupor in filthy gutters only, with the help of those involved in that ministry of healing, to find their way back to health and to undertake a ministry of rescuing other alcoholics from their impending self-destruction. James R. Kok writes of the paradox to be seen in this phenomenon: "Wise prophets in every age observe that God rarely finds people useful to his purposes that have not been broken by life."[2] It may take a large bashing in life to deflate a person's spiritual self-sufficiency. This can lead to the beginning of faith.

Bruce Chilton, rector of a parish in Tarrytown, New York, writing about the importance of losing the personal self in order to gain the God-given self, offers a similar assessment of the purpose of human suffering. "Suffering brings us an awareness of our vulnerability in every sense. It breaks our illusion of control and personal strength. That is the *pain* which is greater than (suffering) *pain*."[3] Through the cross, God gives us the true self, the hope and joy greater than both types of pains.

Saint Paul had such a transformation through suffering in mind. Writing to the Christian community in Rome, he declared to them that "we also boast in our sufferings, knowing that suffering produces endurance, and endurance produces character, and character produces hope, and hope does not disappoint us . . ." (Romans 5:3-5).

The theme of dying to self in order to live a new life in more intimate union with the Spirit of God through our unselfish assistance to those in need is not something new in Judeo-Christian history. Walter J. Burghardt, founding editor of *The Living Pulpit*, echoes this same theme, likening the death to self involved as akin to the death of Jesus. "Dying in a theological sense begins when living begins; we share in Jesus' dying through the whole of our lives."[4] Burghardt goes on to note that pain itself, disappointment, death of a loved one, insecurity, and aging are akin to dying by installments.[5] Here the final cry of Jesus from the cross, "Father, into your hands I commend my spirit" (Luke 23:46), becomes in Luke's Gospel the supreme act of Jesus' affirming eternal life in the face of an inglorious death.

Some famous contemporary figures can likewise serve as sources of hope and inspiration for us all in how to bear with chronic, incurable suffering. Joni Eareckson Tada, Brian Stenberg, and Christopher Reeve, for example, who once were excellent athletes, became models of endurance for the neurologically handicapped. All three became quadriplegic following cervical spinal cord trauma. Now married, Joni, an athlete and an avid skier, dove into shallow water which resulted in her paralysis. Her brokenness has led her to dedicate her life to God, sharing her faith and hope with others. Christopher Reeve, an acclaimed film actor, sustained cord damage following a fall while on horseback. Before his death he had devoted time and talents to promote further research in the field of spinal cord damage. Brian Stenberg, a promising young pole-vaulter, suffered a similar fate by landing on his neck while training on a trampoline. Although recent stem cell research suggests that new spinal cord nerve cells may be able to correct this kind of damage in the future, nonetheless, it remains a mystery why bad things are allowed to happen to such good people. One might speculate that God created all of us to be to be people of faith, to encourage hope, to bring people closer to God, and, perhaps, in the case of this trio of athletes, to push research for new cures. The good that comes out of these tragedies may very well be the heroic gifts of endurance, faith, and hope demonstrated by these handicapped persons inspiring others with severe neurological injuries, and teaching compassion to all of us who may be more fortunate.

Some caregivers are called to be the presence of God in the lives of the chronically ill, offering comfort and healing where possible. Matthew Fox, a former Dominican priest and noted author, commenting on this aspect of his ministry, says that it is his pleasure to be involved in relieving the pain of others, because, as a compassionate Christian, it is his pain and God's pain as well. He states that there is a pressing need to realize that acts of compassion are to everyone's own best interest. Fox believes that this is the highest experience of the spiritual life, and the survival of our planet depends largely on such compassion.[6] In communion with Jesus Christ, who acts vicariously through them, the compassionate presence and healing efforts of health care providers can be redemptive. By being united with the one who suffers, the caregiver is then meeting God in the one who has by illness become one of the least of Jesus' brothers and sisters (see Matthew 25:31-46). In like manner, when a patient is terminal or critically ill, family, friends, clergy, and the entire caretaker team deeply involved in the individual's care will also suffer as they share the burden with the patient and give so much of themselves in caring for the sick and the dying.

DOCTOR BILL'S PERSONAL REFLECTIONS

Every physician will encounter over a lifetime of practice count-less cases of suffering among people living with lethal diseases or other severe and often painful conditions. Although cancers can be palliated or cured, and the same holds true for a host of illnesses, many have died despite our best and most modern treatments. We cannot control all things, and we do not know all the answers. The mission of health caregivers is to be a presence among the sick and dying entrusted to them. We can become the vicarious presence of the God who cares in the final stages of life. This is an awesome respon-sibility and, in the spirit of faith, a privilege. We should acknowledge our willingness to join prayer to our medical ministrations. This can only reinforce the comfort we hope to bring to our healing efforts, not only to those caught in the suffering of their illnesses, but to their loved ones as well.

I will always remember the case of a nineteen-year-old student at Princeton University. Standing in the dormitory room with her room-mates, she suddenly shouted, "O my God!" and collapsed to the floor. Her roommates shouted from the second floor window for help. None of them knew how to perform CPR (cardiopulmonary resuscitation). By the time the proctors responded to the cries of the students and ar-rived at the room, several minutes had passed. The rescue squad was quick to answer the call, but several more minutes had gone by. Her heart revealed a lethal rhythm (ventricular fibrillation); this re-sponded to cardioversion and her blood pressure returned, but her brain function never recovered. The pain was almost unbearable for her family, for the nurses, clergy, and all of us involved in her care. After a myriad of consultations and tests, carried out over several days, the conclusion was reached that her brain had been permanently damaged; the coma persisted and all reflexes had gone. We all held hands at her bedside and prayed as she was allowed to slip away. Her family decided to donate her organs. I feel it is safe to say that a part of everyone there died with her that sad day. In medical practice one can enter in the joy of medical cures, but along with the joy, there will always be the less common and unforgettable case where we experi-ence this kind of overwhelming sadness.

Health caregivers must remember that, in their ministry to their pa-tients, the needs of the patients will always be greater than they can possibly address fully. Even with our best efforts, people will sicken and die. We all die at some point. Even Lazarus, after being raised from the dead, ultimately died. We seem to lose sight of this fact. Perhaps we are in some way denying our own death in struggling vainly to maintain life in a terminally ill patient in the last stages of dying. Our task as health care providers is to do our best for the patient and, depending on our faith, to pray for a healing and thereby continue to be channels for healing the hurts of others. God, however, is the final source of the patient's progress toward health. Healings, even in the case of the restoration to health from an otherwise terminal illness, are but reprieves from the inevitability of death.

THE DECEASED BELOVED AND THE LEGACY LEFT BEHIND

Although attending the death of a patient or a loved one is a painful experience that often brings grief to the health caregiver, I am continually amazed with the many good things that can serve as a legacy upon a person's physical death. In some instances, family members who had been at odds with each other over many years have reconciled at the death of their loved one. The tragedy probably moved them to think seriously about what they should mean to each other, given their common ties of blood and of the love they shared. In some instances, funds for medical research, monies for new and established social service projects have resulted through expressions of sympathy for the loved ones or their families. Organs of a recently deceased person have been donated to those who desperately await them. Likewise, memorial scholarships have been given for talented but poor students. We read that similar gifts have been granted to the children of firefighters who died in the Twin Towers tragedy in New York. We should not lose sight of the fact that although there is a physical death for a given person, the same person lives on in spirit, and can remain with us for years to come. Our faith even tells us of our eventual reunion with the loved ones who have passed the threshold of this life into life everlasting.

The grieving period always follows the death of a loved one. I have noticed that even in cases of longstanding illness (e.g., very elderly patients suffering with a multitude of symptoms), the family caregivers are never quite prepared for the death of the loved one when the time eventually arrives. Emotionally it is a time for a farewell to the physical presence of this person. All that is left are the memories of better times together that have accumulated over the years. The need for grieving in these cases is just as great as in cases in which sudden, unexpected, or premature death of a young person occurs.

TIME WITH THE FAMILY FOLLOWING THE DEATH OF THE BELOVED

I found that in virtually all cases in which a loved one has died, whether it was sudden and unexpected, or following a long illness, it is important for me to set aside time in the office for the immediate family. This time is reserved for easing the minds of those friends or family members involved in that person's care. Normal questions include the cause of death, the choice of treatments given, and whether there was a genetic basis for the illness that could be passed on to other family members, or an infectious cause, such as tuberculosis, AIDS, or hepatitis that might be contagious for the family members. An opportunity is given to try to answer any or all questions or concerns that might be preying on the minds of the family. This is a time for compassion, as the physician listens attentively and responds as best as possible to all the issues of concern. It also is a time to acknowledge the thanks of the family for the medical care that was given. At times the remaining spouse or close family member may be overburdened with false guilt. In my view, it is very important to alleviate this burden and to give ample reassurance that the care given by the family for the loved one was very well done, and that no one could have done better. Certainly, this is true in the overwhelming number of cases. So many times, in hindsight, a family member might regret not having recognized the very early symptoms, or not calling for help sooner, or not being present at the bedside at the exact time of death. "If I had only done this or that" has been repeated at least a thousand times over my career, and each time this only serves to intensify the grief. To see the bereaved person sigh and show a small smile through the veil of tears, and leave the office having been reassured with the words, "No one could have done better," has been one of the most liberating experiences in medicine. A minor miracle occurs when the distraught and dedicated family member is released from this false guilt, to attain a sense of inner peace once again, to return to living once more, and ultimately to be able to celebrate the life of the beloved.

Physicians are taught to treat the ill patient to the best of our abilities. When death finally intervenes, we must not forget those who remain behind, those who must go on living with a free heart, not one burdened with the "what ifs" for the rest of their lives. This is a time of compassion at work. Obviously, all of this cannot be so easily attained, especially at one visit, but it does make a big start in the healing process. Matthew Fox describes compassion as "feelings of togetherness." We are urged to rejoice at another's joy and grieve at another's sorrow. He remarks, "Both dimensions, celebration and sorrow, are integral to true compassion. Compassion is not sentiment but is making justice and doing works of mercy."[7]

A German proverb also speaks to this: "A sorrow shared is a sorrow halved; joy shared is a joy doubled." At times audible prayers can be offered. But an inaudible prayer, consisting of just being present to the family and listening with a sympathetic ear, often is sufficient.

A severe personal loss will likely trigger suffering and pain. This may include the patient's struggle with a terminal illness as well as the pain and suffering on the part of his or her caregiver. We continue to be broken as the years go by, often in small ways as well in deeper ways; this all goes with the turf, and it is part of living. The Lord gave me a good bashing in 1980 when I was not listening to him, too busy to seek his guidance, resulting in my crawling to him for mercy and guidance during my recovery period. This period of suffering became a turning point in my life. God's plan for me was to be more open to the divine love and to express this in my practice and personal life. I am now better able to recognize my own deficiencies in not fully responding to the full range of the needs of others as I continue to learn how to reach out and love others.

PREMONITIONS OF DEATH:
GOD'S PROVIDENTIAL CARE

God may give someone a premonition of his or her impending death. I remember an eight-year-old boy, the son of the roofer for our house, who had always enjoyed good health. He was a physically active child, a member of a Little League baseball team. He was never seriously sick. One day his mother looked over his shoulder and noticed that he was drawing a gravestone with his name on it. She became upset and asked him why he was doing this. He replied, "I'm going to meet Jesus, and *it's going to be all right.*" About a week later, while running from the dugout to the outfield during a game, he suddenly fell over and died. It turned out that he had a rare congenital heart condition that had never been detected. His mother has since remarked that, despite her deep grief, the one thing that has sustained her was remembering her son's words: "It's going to be all right." This gave a considerable peace to the distraught family remembering those words as a prophecy about his seeing Jesus. I cannot help wondering about God inspiring the young boy to write those words with a view to easing the inevitable grief that the family was about to experience. Many times God's actions remain a mystery for us. The boy's younger sister, upon further testing, has inherited the same cardiac abnormality. But in her case the prospects are optimistic with very effective treatments available for the condition once it is recognized. Again, would his sister's incipient problem have been discovered were it not for the death of her brother? God's ways are certainly not our ways.

God, in his own mysterious way, may also provide an unexpected comfort for the person about to die. In one case, I had been making hospital rounds as usual on a morning that could be labeled for us doctors as "a busy day in the marketplace." I was running late and had a busy day awaiting me in the office. My inner voice said, "Go see Helga now." She was a lovely elderly patient of long-standing, receiving chemotherapy under the care of her oncologist for widespread cancer. Often I would try to do a "social call" on a patient who was temporarily being treated by a specialist in a different field than mine. My first response to the inner voice was, "The end of the day would work best for me. I'm already late for the office." The response I sensed was, "No! Go now!"

After going back and forth with this inner dialogue, I finally decided I would give up and listen to the voice and respond. As I entered the room, Helga disarmed me with her warm, friendly manner and remarked how happy she was to see me. She was so delighted to see me and thanked me more than once for stopping by. She was a very spiritual woman and over the years had frequently and quite openly discussed how much God had done for her. We stayed together, holding hands, and having a good conversation. It was truly a prayerful visit. I remember that she looked surprisingly well, considering her diagnosis. Helga stated that she was to be discharged in about four days. As it was mid-April, she could not wait to be with her grandson and do a little work in her garden. After a few more moments of conversation, I told her that I would try to stop by to see her every day until she went home. We waved to each other as I left, and once again she remarked how pleased she was that I had stopped by to see her. About twenty minutes later, when I was in the middle of the office work, the nurse from her floor called and noted that Helga had just peacefully passed away. I learned then how important it is to listen to those inner urgings, even in the busy times of the day, because they are God's voice asking me to be on hand for someone in need of my care. We may speak of how coincidental encounters such as these are. But for me the urge to forget my inconveniences was the voice of God caring for one of his dying children.

AFTER-DEATH EXPERIENCES

Valerie is an example of this phenomenon. Valerie was an eighty-year-old patient who came to the ER complaining of recent fainting spells. After being placed on a monitor, she became unconscious. Her pacemaker failed to capture the ventricle and she suffered cardiac arrest. She was obviously pacemaker-dependent. Fortunately, a temporary external pacemaker was only a few feet away and put to use. Her blood pressure and pulse responded. She became alert again. She had been resuscitated in a matter of minutes. She was given a new pacemaker battery and discharged in two days. Valerie had been "brought back" after her cardiac arrest much to the delight of her daughter and grandchildren. During a subsequent office visit, she described her experience of being in a tunnel and bathed in a warm, pleasant white light. In addition, she noted with great joy the presence of family members who had predeceased her. Upon further reflection, she realized that it was so pleasant that she had wished she had not been resuscitated. She even wrote a letter to me stating both her experience and her frustration about the whole episode.

This kind of experience can become a source of comfort for those of us who are still here. Some critics say the experience may also be due to some biochemical changes occurring in the brain during those near-death situations, perhaps a transient lack of oxygen. Nevertheless, it was a peaceful adventure for her. I like to think that God is there, waiting to greet us along with former friends and family. A wonderful reunion! An increasing number of scientists believe life is a continuum, that there is an afterlife, and that, with physical death, our spirit lives on. I feel the physician needs this kind of confidence when dealing with the terminally ill.

Some believe, too, that our full healing may occur only at death. Kenneth Ring, a professor of psychology at the University of Connecticut, has spent the last twenty years studying near-death experience (NDE). He recorded firsthand accounts of a few hundred people in his book *Heading Toward Omega.* A general consensus among the individuals in the study concerns events that occur when experiencing a NDE.[8] Ring notes the overwhelming peace and joy to be found during this time. During the NDE, individuals are aware of an absence of pain and bodily sensations. Not infrequently, an "out-of-body" experience is described whereby the individual hovers above the physical body, as if the person were a detached spectator to all that is going on in the area. Many describe an increase in both visual and hearing acuity. An awareness of floating, often at a terrific speed inside a dark but peaceful tunnel, has been a rather common experience. Near the end of the NDE, a "presence," not actually seen, stimulates a review of the person's life and then asks whether the individual wants to live or die. The experience quickly ends when the choice to return to earthly life is made.

In some circumstances, the experience is allowed to proceed further before the question is asked. In these cases, the person may float peacefully toward a bright white light that is painless to the eyes, and is warm and welcoming. Others experience a sensation of floating into a "world of light," where they are reunited with those who have died previously. If one is told that it is not yet the time to remain in this state, the person is either commanded or chooses to return to earthly life. Virtually all of those interviewed by Ring describe being enveloped by an environment of pure love, great joy, and compassion when experiencing this dying process. Ring estimates that about 35 to 40 percent of individuals who come close to death undergo a NDE encompassing many of the previously described sensations. Some of the comments made by those individuals included the following:

There was a total immersion in light, in peace, in security, and
warmth.
It was a beautiful white light; it becomes you and you become it.
It was all being, all beauty, all meaning of existence. Love was
all around me.
I was aware . . . of my past life. It was like it was being recorded. . . . There was the warmest, most wonderful love, Love all
around me . . . I felt light-good-happy-joy-at ease. Forever—
eternal love. Time meant nothing. Just being. Love. Pure love.[9]

Following a death, many writers have experienced the nearness of
the former loved one guiding and blessing them. At times I have mentioned that I sense my parents' spiritual nearness as they send their
love and guidance to me and my family. They desire to send their
prayers to us, and likely need our prayers as well. George A. Maloney
makes the point that our loved ones in heaven continue to receive both
Christ's love and our love; they are thereby released from their hurts
and set free to love us in return, and more deeply than when they were
present with us on earth.

How often I feel united with my departed father! How often I
felt his loving intercession for me! Persons who have lost loved
ones have often reported to me how present they are to their beloved ones . . . Can anyone guarantee that when the departed
ones are loved in Christ, they cannot return that love by sharing
a protective hand.[10]

GEFF'S THEOLOGICAL REFLECTION
ON SUFFERING, DEATH, AND GRIEF

In his book *Recovering from the Losses of Life,* H. Norman Wright
mentions that our work of grieving is not really done until we discover a meaning in this process. We have a need for an inner healing as well as a healing of our system of beliefs and our theology.[11]
"Why did God let this happen?" can be a very difficult question to answer. Paul's taunt to death in his letter to the Christians of Corinth,
"Where, O death, is your victory? Where, O death, is your sting?"

(1 Corinthians 15:55) is often invoked to bolster the boast of Christians that they do not or should not fear death. However, for most people, death has never lost its "sting" and the fear of death and its prelude of suffering is still very much with us.

Evelyn Underhill reminds us in her study of mysticism that "pain plunges like a sword through creation."[12] Even Jesus had to pass "through a labyrinth of many woes,"[13] before entering into the glory that the Hebrew scriptures declare is due the just person who dies serving God. For Christians, Christ's suffering offers, not escape from the sorrows of life, but an exemplary source of meaning in which one's own sufferings can open up possibilities in which one's weakness or illness can be accepted and even welcomed as a new challenge and a source of comfort and encouragement.

Not everyone can accept these challenges or even appreciate the biblically based alleviation of suffering offered by Jesus in the Gospels and proclaimed by Paul in his letters. I entered that reality during my daughter's long struggle with the brain tumor that threatened her life. When she was undergoing chemotherapy over a period of two years, I began a support group to help parents share stories and frustrations, thus helping one another cope with the agony of watching our children being subjected to the painful needles and poisonous chemicals in the hospital's inexorable protocol of treatments. Among the fourteen parents, only two were men. What shocked me, though, was the admission by six of the women that their husbands had left them, unable to bear the difficulties of attending to the needs of a sick or dying child or the loss of intimacy in their marriage. As one mother put it bluntly: "It was pretty hard to make love while our daughter was suffering in the next bedroom." I realized that catastrophic illness does not always bring out the best in people; nor does it always draw families closer together. As one writer remarked, quoting a then separated couple: "It's like our lives were supposed to end up in Southern California and we got hijacked to the Arctic Circle!"[14]

Pain and suffering are not necessarily redemptive or even guaranteed not-to-fail boosters for our practice of compassion for others who may be trapped in the fellowship of debilitating illness, sudden loss of strength or life, and grief for one's own misery and that of others. Nor can we say that those who have drawn on their own sufferings as motivation and energizer in their compassion and in the generous help they are able to give others, were themselves without moments of anger, resentment, and pleas for redress. Through the grace of God that came in many forms, including the personal presence and support of others, they were able to bring their wounded inner resources to the surface for healing.

JESUS' COURAGE IN THE FACE OF SUFFERING

The self-inflicted pain idealized in many saints and ascetics of old was destined to give way to a spirit of acceptance of and resignation to whatever God permitted to happen to us in a world where the weakest and most vulnerable people are made to suffer at the hands of domineering, malevolent powers. Jesus is now considered by many theologians the innocent victim of heartless religious leaders and the cruel oppressors sent by imperial Rome. His stolid faith showed Christians the redemptive value of suffering for others. Robert Morris called Jesus' amazing calm before his accusers and executioners the "midnight sky" rooted in his heart. Jesus was able to focus, not on the dangers of the moment, but on the vast wonder of the starry skies created and maintained by his Father God. In Morris's words:

> Then I inwardly saw Jesus standing silently before Pilate, and realized that the midnight sky was in his heart. He was not standing passively accepting abuse, but nobly, without fear, facing his enemy with courage and compassion, *because he was rooted in a goodness deeper than the suffering.* Even in the midst of suffering, the taproot of his spirit was deeply anchored in the goodness of God. I realized in that moment that this was Jesus' secret of facing life in this wild, wonderful, and terribly difficult universe.[15]

The Gospels are clear in claiming that Jesus was never trapped in the pit of his own sufferings, buoyed up, as he was, by the overriding confidence of knowing that God's indestructible love was alive within him. He was, in short, a bearer of God's presence even in the darkest corners of the world where disease, enmities, violence, and death lurked. Jesus' bravery was but an echo of God's own power in inspiring people to courageously unmask the causes of human suffering and to offer their own graced potential to alleviate in their ministries the sorrows that ensue when God's way of love is rejected and the innocent suffer.

Jesus' example became a inspiration to Dietrich Bonhoeffer in his own struggles to deliver his nation and the world from the horrors of a world at war and the daily murders in the death camps of Nazi Germany. Those who opposed the Hitlerian tyranny had many grim prospects to face. Theirs was a lonely battle against their own government. Few would consider their opposition to Nazism as anything but disloyalty and a lack of patriotism. Nonetheless, they could look on the sufferings of Jesus in order to bolster their spirits in those moments when discouragement could set in and the noose of the Gestapo drawn ever more tightly around them in their conspiracy. Hence, he wrote an essay letter to his fellow resisters as a Christmas present of encouragement while they were preparing the first of several failed attempts to overthrow the government by assassinating Hitler. Bonhoeffer wrote:

> It is infinitely easier to suffer in obedience to a human command than in the freedom of one's own responsibility. It is infinitely easier to suffer with others than to suffer alone. It is infinitely easier to suffer publicly and honorably than apart and ignominiously. It is infinitely easier to suffer through staking one's life than to suffer spiritually. Christ suffered as a free man alone, apart and in ignominy, in body and spirit; and since then many Christians have suffered with him.[16]

The mystery of suffering brings together, then, both those who suffer and those who minister to them. Two dynamics converge as the caregiver and the one who suffers enter into a fellowship with each other. No facile theological or ascetical formula exists for the healing of one's ills, whether physical or emotional. The old counsel that I learned early on in my religious training was "to offer it up." We were told that such sacrifice of our normal feelings was a rich source of grace that could even be applied to others more in need of God's grace. Some examples:

> I don't like what that person did to me, but I offer it up for my Uncle Louie who is a hopeless drunk. Please help him, Lord.

I'd really like to punch that nasty person in the nose, but I offer it up for the souls in purgatory.

I'm sick as a dog, but I offer my illness up to help convert some lost soul.

If we believe in the central Jewish belief that we are all created in God's image, the connection is far from tenuous. Nor do we live on isolated islands, as the poet John Donne reminds us. Paul even tells us that, contrary to the popular attitude toward suffering, he actually rejoices in his sufferings for the sake of his Christians because in his "flesh [he is] completing what is lacking in Christ's afflictions for the sake of his body, that is, the church" (Colossians 1:24).

SUFFERING AS A PATH TO HOLINESS

But there is much more to suffering than the possible benefits of one's self-sacrifices. Suffering is for some a path toward a holiness that may have eluded them during their lifetimes. The path to empathy for another's troubles is often strewn with the tears that persons have shed during their own dark evenings of enduring pain and physical or emotional distress. Henri Nouwen speaks of the "wounded healer,"[17] implying that a healer often has to pass through that vale of personal sorrow in order to be a helpful presence to others who are crying out for relief from their misery.

Ginger Grab points out that Shakespeare's drama of King Lear offers a salutary lesson in the power of suffering to provoke a conversion. The impulsive, arrogant Lear, when "sane," could not see his insane rage as anything other than normal. But once awakened from his madness and his addiction to the domineering attitudes that had ruined his life, he experiences a liberation from his destructive past. Now he can recognize that all the trappings of his kingship had only eroded his true nature as a vulnerable human being. He is freed from the senseless bondage to his self-centeredness and the hatred it had spawned. He is freed to love again. In Grab's words: "He loses the world and gains his soul."[18]

However, not everyone's soul is rescued by suffering. Suffering with patience can instill unexpected power to soften a person's diffidence toward the sufferings of others and possibly incline those who have suffered to become compassionate healers themselves. Rabbi Harold Kushner likes to tell the old Chinese story about a grieving woman and a magical mustard seed.

The woman's only son had died and so she sought out the holy man to ask for a set of prayers or some magical incantations to bring her son back to life. Instead of remonstrating with the woman he sent her on the "quest" that would bring her son back. She was to fetch him "a mustard seed from a home that has never known sorrow. We will use it to drive the sorrow out of your life." Everywhere she went, whether to a stately mansions, a palace, or the hovels of the poor, looking for the home that had never known sorrow, she met people who all had sad stories of their personal tragedies. She stayed to offer them comfort because she understood how her own sorrow had torn her life apart. She became so involved in consoling these grieving people that unconsciously she drove her own sorrowing and self-pity from her heart and no longer needed to look for that magical mustard seed.[19]

Rabbi Kushner uses the story to point out that those we might envy for their success or their wealth or their seeming happiness may have personal problems and histories of sorrow that are well hidden from us.

GOD'S PRESENCE AMID OUR SUFFERING

In all of our attempts to reach out to comfort the sorrowing, however, there is for many the sustaining force that comes with living in the presence of God. With God there is no pretense. God sees us as we are and bids us to do the same and discover the possibilities for healing the troubles of others through our own compassion. Our presence in consoling those in sorrow and grief will not take away their hurt. Short of successful medical intervention, we will not cure their illness. Nor can we bring back their loved ones to life. And, even less, will we offer them the solution to the perennial question of why God permits such suffering in the first place. As New Testament scholar David Rensberger points out, what we can offer them may be simply the message of the cross:

Not that God will shield us from suffering, but that we can encounter God in our suffering, even as God has encountered us in human suffering. God knows our suffering. Coming into God's presence as sufferers, we can learn who we are, in our suffering and beyond suffering, and we can learn who God is, the God who suffers and the God who both transcends and transforms suffering.[20]

Such a transformation is never predictable. For Rabbi Kushner the transformation is not found in coming up with pat theological answers to why people suffer but in acknowledging that God does, indeed, sorrow with us in our sorrows, and that God is wounded in those wanton acts when evil is done to the innocent. God's presence to relieve suffering is discovered in the presence of those who seem sent to us as God's emissaries of consolation and support. God, in mysterious ways, ultimately gives the grace to cope with suffering and to extend our gracious help to others. In Rabbi Kushner's words:

> God does not want you to be sick or crippled. He didn't make you have this problem, and he doesn't want you to go on having it, but he can't make it go away. That is something which is too hard even for God. What good is he, then? God makes people become doctors and nurses to try to make you feel better. God helps us be brave even when we're sick and frightened, and he reassures us that we don't have to face our fears and our pains alone.[21]

Rabbi Kushner is adamant that God's gift of freedom puts God in a bind not to intervene when the laws set to govern nature and health are violated. The bullet that kills has neither rationality nor conscience; the bombs of the terrorist or the smart military bombs gone astray do not respect the goodness of those killed or the feelings of their loved ones. God's creation is a work of beauty and complexity; his creation is flawed and even chaotic in order to make freedom and love possible.

DEALING WITH DEATH AND GRIEF

If suffering is inevitable, so too is death and the grief people experience when a loved one dies. At this juncture, pious words or spiritual bromides will never lessen the pain or provide the healing that those lost in their grief need.

Rabbi Kushner likens the religious prattle, intended to soften or explain away the sorrow of losing a loved one, to the annoying intrusions on Job's grief by his friends.[22] God does help and the scriptures do offer comfort, but all in their proper time and properly understood. The grieving need sympathy, not explanatory sermons. They need the presence of compassionate friends who can tolerate their emotional upset, outbursts, and tears. This solace, Rabbi Kushner argues, is what religion does best. It provides a community of support where people can be caring and where the grieving can know they are not alone in their sorrow. In Rabbi Kushner's words: "God, who neither causes nor prevents tragedies, helps by inspiring people to help."[23] For those who have experienced suffering and grief he asks that they find it in their hearts to forgive God for this less-than-perfect world and for all the disappointments, sickness, and cruelty that are the dark downside of our freedom.

He asks further that people "recognize that the ability to forgive and the ability to love are the weapons God has given us to enable us to live fully, bravely, and meaningfully in this less-than-perfect world."[24] Rabbi Kushner admits that his own attitudes toward suffering and death have been inspired by the heroic struggle of his son, Aaron, against the progeria disease that took his life at a very young age. Rabbi Kushner speaks with the authority of one who has traversed that same valley of darkness with countless others of his congregation and later of the much wider world who have read his books and heard his talks. He has helped those struggling with grief in their personal tragedies through his stories of compassion and probing questions into the possible meaning of human suffering and death in a world obviously not under the tight-fisted control of an all-powerful deity.

VARYING ATTITUDES TOWARD DEATH:
RELIGIOUS INSIGHTS

Attitudes toward death vary from acceptance to denial with several emotions in between, some of which range from joy in being delivered from pain, fear at not knowing where one is headed after death, to sorrow at having to leave one's loved ones behind. The Bible speaks of not fearing evil while walking "through the darkest valley" (Psalm 23:4), or living in the shadow of death because the Lord is there to lead us and protect us. For Gerald Janzen, this Psalm does not really remove fear but it does assist us to face that fear by unmasking death's pretension to be the ultimate reality of our lives. He acknowledges his own personal anxiety, but denies

> its claim to be ultimate in my life and in the world. It may mug me or take me hostage in whatever dark valley of grief, depression, oppression, or other trouble I may be passing through. It may even kill me. But in the face of that evil and the fear it evokes I will affirm the ultimacy of God.[25]

Janzen's strong belief in the ultimate reality beyond death dovetails well with the theology of death of the Jesuit scholar, Karl Rahner. Similar to Janzen, Rahner is equally insistent that the lesson of death is that death will never have the last word, but that death itself is only the prelude to the beginning of a new life with God.

> Throughout all of the words of scripture we always surmise one and the same thing: God is absolute mystery. And therefore fulfillment and absolute closeness to God himself is also an ineffable mystery which we go to meet and which the dead who die in the Lord find, as the Apocalypse says. It is the mystery of ineffable happiness. It is no wonder, then, that our ears do not hear the pure silence of this happiness."[26]

These are words of hope that one can find in the scriptural assurances that God has prepared wondrous blessings for those who love God, such as human eyes have not seen nor ears heard or even entered in our hearts, as Paul exclaimed in his praise of God's wisdom (1 Corinthians 2:9).

Karl Rahner's prayer in which he envisaged his own encounter with death is not unlike Paul's declaration to the Philippians that the joy of being reunited with Jesus Christ outweighs all fear of his impending execution (Philippians 1:20-23). Rahner is convinced that his death will transcend all human words.

> I will know as I am known, will understand what you have always said to me, namely yourself. No human word, no image and no concept will ever stand between me and you; you yourself will be

the one joyful word of love and life that fills all the spheres of my soul.[27]

Rahner's anticipation of eternal life in the face of death and his never ceasing proclamation of God's goodness and the holy mystery of God's infinite love for his creatures helps us understand the vehemence with which he denounced Augustine's preaching of "massa damnata" [the damned masses—more bluntly, "most people are damned!"], his conviction that, considering the evil of his times and the infection of the human will's power to resist sin, most people were damned.[28] In Rahner's view few, if any, would be "damned."[29]

DEATH AND THE AFTERLIFE

Fear of hell fire is not the worthiest of motives for putting one's affairs in order while living out one's last allotted days in terminal illness. Today the prospect of one's death often brings on the anxiety of not knowing what lies ahead, the mystery of eternal life beyond this life, and of course the sadness of a departure from one's loved ones that appears on the surface at least to last forever. Death is never easy to accept, but the moment of death is eased somewhat by the assurances of the scriptures, particularly those passages that speak of the death and resurrection of Jesus Christ and the death of the innocent, the prayerful intercessions of family and friends, and the presence of loved ones to comfort and embrace. All these ministrations are enhanced by the skilled help of hospice caregivers and the professional assistance of physicians, who are themselves people of compassion tuned into the spiritual dimensions of life and death. Some die peacefully as if in sleep; some die with a struggle; some die violently; some die quickly in tragic accidents—death, as is said from ordinary wisdom, is no respecter of persons. Woody Allen's quip is not out of place: "I don't fear death; I just don't want to be around when it happens!"

After one class in which I described Rahner's theology of death and offered some corroborating passages of consolation from Saint Paul, I was approached by a student who had rostered me for three of his religion courses and whose athletic career in soccer I had followed. He told me that his mother had had a recurrence of cancer and that she was terminally ill with little chance of living beyond the next six months. He asked if I would be willing to talk with her since she was terribly saddened by the thought of her impending death and leaving all her children and grandchildren behind. Her husband had died suddenly several years before. I agreed to meet with her and to speak with her anytime on the telephone. We did arrange a meeting which, despite my apprehension (What could I possibly say to her?), turned out to be very pleasant. I read some passages from the scriptures and reflected on them with her. I shared with her my own experiences of dealing with my daughter who only years before had been declared terminally ill, and I told her about Rahner's theology of death, and, of course, a couple of stories about those who had died, some peacefully, some heroically, some offering inspiration to many others. She was eager to read anything I had on the experience of death. I had no answers, just reflections, prayers, and stories. I gave her my telephone number and said she could phone me any time she felt anxious and we could talk or just pray together.

The book *Tuesdays with Morrie: An Old Man, A Young Man, and Life's Greatest Lesson* had not yet been published. Later, having read the book, I wished I had had it in hand to offer Mary. When I read in that book Morrie's telling Mitch, his friend and former student, about how horrible it was to watch his body slowly deteriorate but suddenly added, "But it's also wonderful because of all the time I get to say good-bye." He then smiled and said: "Not everyone is so lucky." Mitch's surprise at those words came out in his next comment: "Did he really say lucky?"[30] Gratitude for the time she had was also one of the aspects of Mary's lingering illness that she too appreciated, an opportunity to take her leave while she was still lucid. Later we would talk about the reunion with those same loved ones at the time of their own resurrection.

One story I shared with Mary, which made both of us very teary, was told to me after one of my evening lectures at a Catholic parish in Exton. My topic was Dietrich Bonhoeffer's *The Cost of Discipleship*, and what this spiritual classic meant for living the Christian life with integrity. During my talk I could not help but notice a middle-aged man sitting up front who seemed to follow my every word with uncommon avidity—I am used to some of the bored looks my students give me whenever the theology gets too heavy for them. Inevitably I looked mostly at him while I spoke; his obvious interest and attention were reassuring to me. I was thinking: *Well, at least one parishioner was pleased with what I had to say.* After the talk and during the tea, coffee, and cookies, he sought me out to tell me his story. He said he was a traveling salesman who was the incarnation of those traveling salesman jokes. He was married and, during his sales trips, he would typically cheat on his wife and children. He had seven children; the youngest, a five-year-old, had leukemia. When he was home after a particularly successful business trip, his wife asked him to sit that night with their critically ill son who had been hospitalized and not expected to recover. She, who had been at the hospital all day, would then be free to tend to their other children.

As he continued to tell his story tears streamed down his face.

> All of a sudden, he said, my son who had been asleep sat up in bed. He reached out his arms and called to me, "Daddy, Daddy, it's so beautiful; come and see. It's so beautiful!" and reaching out his arms he fell back on the pillow and died. There seemed to be a light in the room hovering over him. I got down on my knees and begged God to forgive me all my sins and asked him to take care of my son whom I had neglected. My heart was broken and yet I felt closer to my son than I had ever been. Ever since, on all my trips I remain faithful to my wife; I find a church in which to pray, or a priest or minister with whom I can chat, or this evening a religious talk I can go to. That's why I came here tonight. I owe my life, my marriage, my love of Jesus, to my dead son. I read the Bible. I pray whenever I can. When I die I'll be with my son again.

It was obvious from his tears that he must often relive that moment when his son went toward the beauty that is God. I had no words for him, just my own tears, and thanks for his sharing a very moving story with me. Later when my own daughter was near death, I recalled his words and was strengthened for what then seemed our inevitable loss and her release from suffering. Mary, too, would go toward that beauty everlasting. She died very peacefully not long after that meeting. Mary was surrounded by her family. I hoped in my heart during the Mass of the Resurrection that she too had seen that beauty just before breathing her last.

DEATH AS A "FRIEND"

Experiences such as these tend to lighten the burden of death and grief that can otherwise be overwhelming. The film *Tuck Everlasting* reinforces what is often taken for granted in death, namely, that it is a necessary aspect of life, the capstone of a life well lived, and even at times, the occasion to retroactively redeem a life not well spent, as in the case of Tolstoy's *Death of Ivan Ilyich.* In the film, as in the book, the Tuck family is blessed (or doomed) with eternal life after drinking from a magic spring in a thick forest. They cannot die; they cannot be killed. The young Winnie Foster discovers their secret; in the film, she falls in love with the youngest Tuck, Jesse. She is also exposed to the downside of living forever. One son, Miles, has lost his wife and children; his wife had been frightened away by his never aging. He outlived his children and saw their deterioration. The Tucks were hounded because they seemed to be in league with evil spirits. In the film, once he saw the love between Jesse and Winnie begin to blossom, Tuck senior explained to Winnie that she needed to know what life without death was like. Those so doomed became like rocks never changing, so unlike the seasons and the flow of nature. "Don't be afraid of death, Winnie," he said. "Be afraid of the unlived life." In the book, Tuck senior's words of wisdom are just as forceful:

> But dying's part of the wheel [of life], right there next to being born. You can't pick out the pieces you like and leave the rest. Being part of the whole thing, that's the blessing. But it's passing us by, us Tucks. Living's heavy work, but off to one side, the way *we* are, it's useless, too. It don't make sense. If I knowed how to climb back on the wheel, I'd do it in a minute. You can't have living without dying. So you can't call it living, what we got.[31]

Tuck's advice is not unlike Morrie Schwartz's comment:

> Dying is only one thing to be sad over, Mitch. Living unhappily is something else. So many of the people who come to visit me are unhappy. . . . I may be dying, but I'm surrounded by loving, caring souls. How many people can say that?[32]

In the end Winnie does not join the Tucks but chooses to live a normal life with its cycles of growth, decline, and eventual death. She dies at the age of seventy-eight, before she could be reunited with the Tucks and her once beloved Jesse. (The film takes some liberties with the book.)

The death of Joseph Cardinal Bernardin offered all of America the example of how a saintly priest faced his dying with equanimity. In addition to the documentary on his life,[33] we are able to read of his personal reactions to the terminal illness that was killing him through his book *The Gift of Peace*. Nearly every step in his progressive physical deterioration is covered as Bernardin shared his personal story with his people, even the frustrating details of his struggle with pancreatic cancer. He speaks of suffering in communion with Jesus Christ and of his newfound ministry as "unofficial chaplain" to fellow cancer patients during his recovery periods. His visits to the hospital for chemotherapy became also visits to other patients who were going through a similar ordeal. He called this phase of his life a "life-giving ministry" in which he admitted that he found himself "time and again being inspired by the bravery and deep faith of others who shared similar battles with cancer."[34] Finally, on learning that his cancer had spread and that his prognosis was not favorable to his survival, he ceased all treatment. In announcing this decision, he was able to tell his fellow priests and his people that, with the strength of the Lord Jesus, he now looked on death as a friend.

> But notice that Jesus did not promise to take away our burdens. He promised to help us carry them. And if we let go ourselves— and our own resources—and allow the Lord to help us, we will be able to see death not as an enemy or a threat but as a friend.[35]

With his life ebbing away he was able to write a letter to his people telling them to "know that I will carry each of you in my heart! Ultimately, we will all be together, intimately united with the Lord Jesus whom we love so much."[36]

These dying thoughts of Cardinal Bernardin are likewise reminiscent of the inspiring farewell letter that Dietrich Bonhoeffer wrote from prison to his best friend, Eberhard Bethge:

> It is certain that we can claim nothing for ourselves, and may yet pray for everything; it is certain that our joy is hidden in

suffering, and our life in death; it is certain that in all this we are in a fellowship that sustains us. In Jesus God has said Yes and Amen to it all, and that Yes and Amen is the firm ground on which we stand.[37]

When we speak of suffering and death in this book, it is with the mixed feelings we have of having been caregivers to those undergoing the pains of chronic illness. We have experienced the joy and heartache of assisting people both in ministering to them in their suffering and assisting them in the last moments of their life before their entering into that new beginning, which is resurrection.

DISCUSSION QUESTIONS

1. Comment on the assertion that the problem of suffering yields no easy answers. What exactly does unexpected suffering teach us?
2. Can the shock of an unexpected debilitating illness or personal loss free us to reevaluate our lives and life's meaning? Explain.
3. Comment on the passage in Luke's Gospel where Jesus' final cry from the cross becomes Jesus' affirming eternal life in the face of a horrible death.
4. Why is it important in health care to remember that the needs of the patients will always be greater than health care providers can possibly address? Apply this to terminal illness and death.
5. In this chapter there are several stories of the death of a patient and of the process of preparing for the death of a patient. Which do you find the most impressive and why?
6. Why is it natural in bearing with a debilitating illness, death, and grief that one experiences moments of anger and resentment? How can a health care provider help people cope with these emotions?
7. How do Jesus' example and teachings help us face suffering with courage and hope?
8. What insight about death can we learn from the stories of Morrie, Mary, and *Tuck Everlasting*?
9. Is suffering a possible path to holiness and wholeness? Explain.
10. Comment on the story of Cardinal Bernardin and the lessons we can learn from his faith-filled death.

Chapter 6

Forgiveness and Reconciliation in the Healing Process

THEOLOGIAN GEFF'S WEDDING GIFT: A MESSAGE OF FORGIVENESS

When Joan and I were married in 1978, my closest friend and co-author of two of my books, Burton Nelson, sent us as a wedding gift a beautifully framed excerpt from Dietrich Bonhoeffer's wedding sermon from prison enhanced by the superb calligraphy of Burton's daughter, Ingrid. However, when I read the quotation I was disappointed; I had expected something more euphoric for the joy of the occasion. It read:

> Live together in the forgiveness of your sins, for without it no human community, least of all a marriage, can survive. Don't insist on your rights, don't blame each other, don't judge or condemn each other, don't find fault with each other, but accept each other as you are, and forgive each other every day from the bottom of your hearts.[1]

The insistence on "every day forgiveness" is what got to me. At the time I could not imagine moments when "forgiveness" would be called for. I was marrying someone who in my eyes was perfectly loveable in every way. Well, she might have to forgive me my own faults, but never would I have to forgive her! Nonetheless we hung the calligraphy in our bedroom. Not long into our marriage those words finally penetrated my consciousness and I realized that the essence of a loving relationship had to include mutual forbearance and forgiveness. Dr. Bill received similar advice. He remembers that when he and Aline were married in 1984, the priest remarked that there are

Is There a God in Health Care?
doi:10.1300/5554_06

three things to remember in every relationship: "forgive; forgive; and forgive!"

Bonhoeffer's words have been a daily reminder of how we can keep our love alive and heal the little hurts that are part of any relationship. In his own life Bonhoeffer saw his nation deteriorate under the drumbeats of hatred and military vengeance orchestrated by Adolf Hitler and the malicious Nazi ideology. He knew firsthand the power of hate for destroying lives. He also insisted in his sermons on the need to practice forgiveness of enemies in the face of a national policy of vindictiveness.

RECONCILIATION AND HEALING

A vital interconnection exists between reconciliation through forgiveness and healing. According to the English theologian Michael Buckley, such reconciliation restores our relationship with God, our neighbors, as well as ourselves.[2] The healing that ensues enables us to live out this restored relationship to its fullest extent as followers of Jesus Christ. The goal of healing is wholeness, so that the one who is physically ill, mentally stressed, or even spiritually weak can be made strong in mind, body, and spirit.

Both reconciliation and healing, therefore, are copartners that play essential roles in the healing process for all people. The vicissitudes of life lead to our being constantly wounded in one way or another; there will always be the need for healing of those wounds. But there are different types of wounds, and clearly not all these impact the patient in the same manner. Although therapies can be directed primarily to the major source of an illness, whether it is spiritual, emotional, or physical, we cannot forget that every illness has an influence on a broader front, encompassing in more than one way, the whole person. For example, a fractured hip has an impact not only upon the physical body, it also touches the individual's emotions and spiritual health as well.

Healing of the *soul,* or inner healing, has its center around the forgiveness of sins. With an attitude of forbearance of others despite their personal flaws and even their sins, and by the grace of God, we are given the power to forgive ourselves as well as others. The inner healing fostered by an attitude of forgiveness also deals with the *emotions* such as anxiety, guilt, unjustified fear, and anger. Successful therapies often require integrating both spiritual as well as emotional conditions in the healing process. Healing of the body pertains to issues that may have originated in or happened to one's emotional state as well as one's physical body. Only the rare illness in the practice of medicine does not have widespread influence on the person's entire physical, spiritual, and emotional makeup.

Our spirituality serves as an anchor for not only the individual's wholeness, but also for the wholeness needed in a community of believers. An individual cannot grow into wholeness by remaining alone. Our nature is interdependent. We cannot survive in isolation; we all need a community in order to grow. We must love and be loved and supported by others as we journey along life paths of return to our creator God.

COMPASSION AND FORGIVENESS
IN THE SERVICE OF HEALING:
DOCTOR BILL'S REFLECTIONS

Many renowned healers speak not only of their empowerment by God to help others but also of their need for them to undergo their own healing in order to be more effective witnesses to the love of God at the heart of healing the hurts of others. Paul Tournier, a Swiss internist and Christian, realized this some sixty years ago: "What we can do for others and for the world at large," he wrote, "must always begin in ourselves. Christian revolution always goes deeper than any ideological revolution because its roots are in a change of heart."[3] The implications of this "revolution" lie in the way our own "change of heart" can lead us to be forgiving of the faults of others and advocates for reconciliation and peace where vengeance-seeking and wars seem to dominate the policies of so many societies in today's world. Lessons in peacemaking can be learned from those pockets of genuine Christian living where daily prayer, forbearance, and forgiveness of sins are the order of the day.

Several years ago my wife, Aline, and I saw the integration of these important dynamics of Christian living firsthand during our visit to the Taizé monastic community. This is an ecumenical monastery in France. During one of his talks with us Brother Roger, the founder of

Taizé, emphasized the virtue of beholding the spirit of God within us in addition to the virtues of forgiveness, compassion, and reconciliation that need to be applied in our world today. His words were unforgettable: "If you remain unforgiving, if you refuse a reconciliation, what do you reflect of Christ? If you lose the ability to forgive, you have lost everything."[4] Brother Roger has also offered a prayer that asks of Jesus the gift of looking toward him at every moment. "So often we forget that you live within us, that you are praying within us, that you are loving within us. Your miracle in us is your trust and your forgiveness, always offered in that unique communion which is called the Church."[5] As I reread those words, I can see more clearly their interconnectedness in the healing profession that has been my lifelong ministry. These are the very virtues coalescing in the love and spirit of forbearance that Jesus declared to be the sign of genuine Christian discipleship.

The connection between forgiveness and healing was brought home to me in a striking way when I was treating Emma in the hospital on a Sunday morning. Emma was a seventy-eight-year-old woman dying from cancer. She was in constant pain and had become bedridden. Her two daughters had not spoken to each other in several years. This problem greatly disturbed Emma and aggravated her condition. When I entered the room I could sense considerable tension in the air. I did not know what the cause of this tension might be. It occurred to me that perhaps a healing prayer would be helpful. I asked everyone present if they would like to join me in a healing prayer for Emma and, of course, for all of us present. The special duty nurse, the two daughters, Emma's husband, and I laid hands on Emma and prayed for God's healing. At the conclusion of the prayer, Emma sighed as if a burden were removed from her chest and the two daughters rushed across the room in tears to hug each other. Seeing her daughters reconciled at last, Emma then experienced an inner calm, less anxiety, and a much more peaceful state of mind. She required less pain medication and slept better. Emma died peacefully a few days later. A spiritual healing had taken place. The two daughters likewise experienced great peace through reconciling their differences during Emma's final days. The stresses that had built up between them were gone. They remain a loving family to this day, something I attribute to the power of prayer. Even though Emma was not cured of her cancer, nonetheless, she and her daughters experienced a remarkable spiritual healing. It was clear to me that somehow we had witnessed the healing presence of God as Emma was being welcomed into her heavenly home.

REJECTION AND THE MINISTRY
OF RECONCILIATION

What is there in one's spiritual makeup that enables genuine healers to withstand burdens of rejection within themselves and to lift these burdens from others? When one has been rejected, a truckload of pain and suffering can easily enter into one's heart. The late Henri Nouwen, a priest and well-known author of books on spirituality, declares that "self-rejection is the greatest enemy to the spiritual life."[6] Nouwen believes that the greatest hindrance to wholeness in our life is not power and wealth; it is the feeling that each of us may become a "nobody," with nothing to offer—one who is rejected. Loneliness is, likewise, one of society's most painful wounds. As Christians we are obligated to seek out our neighbors who are suffering and all alone. Loneliness and pain are often bound together, and this can often be seen when the family unit disintegrates because of death or divorce.

How can we as health caregivers of others handle rejection in ourselves and the pain of rejection in those we are trying to help regain emotional stability? To begin, we can realize that, despite our feelings of inadequacy, we remain in God's love and the Holy Spirit's guidance. We may need to ingrain this thought daily into our hearts. As paradoxical and ironic as it seems, the experience of rejection and brokenness can often lead us to greater intimacy with God and condition us to be more understanding of the turbulence experienced by others. From his own personal experience, Nouwen once remarked, "Just as bread needs to be broken in order to be given, so too, do our lives."[7] Nouwen felt that everything can radically change from the moment we realize that that each of us has been sent into this world to live a life acknowledging that we are chosen by God for a particular ministry. If we are broken here on earth, it is in order to be given in service for others who have experienced their own brokenness.

ISOLATION AND INDIVIDUALISM:
BARRIERS AGAINST RECONCILIATION

The problem of promoting an inner healing through forbearance, forgiveness, and reconciliation is compounded by the way contemporary society has encouraged isolation, rugged individualism, and aggressive self-assertion over others. "Survival of the fittest" and "get a jump on the competition" are common motivational slogans in today's competitive market. These ideas encourage the attitude of thinking of other people as mere stepping-stones to personal success. The paths to this success are marked by reliance on a more aggressive self, making the quick dollar, and the importance of being "number one," whether it is in politics, business, or one's personal life. Not to be highlighted is the reality that, even in the enjoyment of what may be hailed as the successful life by the judges of who ranks where in the ladder of societal success stories, no one is immune from life's hurts and losses. If we truly need to belong to a community of believers for giving and receiving love and support when personal suffering intrudes into one's life, we may ask to whom do the self-confident, self-reliant persons turn to, when they feel overwhelmed by tragic turns in their family and career plans? Personal suffering may be further complicated by the fact that today's neighbors come and go; there are more frequent changes in job locations now than twenty-five years ago. A community of believers located in a certain neighborhood may move to another state a few years later. How does one promote peace and reconciliation in today's society if the prevailing attitude is to look out only for oneself and to ignore those who might disturb our peace by pressing their needs on us?

Our society is such that often people do not know those who live next door. We have become strangers and in many cases we have lost our neighborliness. Even lifetime friends may move away or die. Some of society's fragmentation can be traced to broken homes, and "downsizing" with loss of jobs. Our culture is hurting in many areas: character assassination against candidates for public office, destruction of open space, the loss of farms through progressive urban sprawl. Children have fewer role models as they watch violence overdone in the TV news, movies, and video games. Insurance companies have invaded the practice of medicine, the primary concern being the bottom line rather than the well-being of the patient in a number of cases.

We might ask some serious questions in the face of these harsh realities: Why has anxiety replaced inner peace? Where is the respect for the "nonproductive" elderly? Perhaps most important: how do we expect to raise children in our current cynical, violence-condoning, and materialistic environment?

Given the contemporary frenetic pace of life, we need a societal healing turnabout, a moral and spiritual revolution. Although individuals in our culture turn to God in times of loss or great stress and request rescue and healing, such as in the aftermath of the Columbine shootings, or the events of September 11, 2001, it is doubtful many relied upon God *before* those terrible things happened. Will we continue to be isolated and self-reliant? Gary Ross, writer and movie director, reflecting on his goals and motivations, stated that, given society's malaise, he will ask himself the question in all future screenplays, "what the ramifications are to the culture in which I live and the children who may see these films." He also lists a number of negative factors that are unhealthy for today's society in the U.S.:

- A decrease in a sense of security, a decrease in job performance, or loss of close personal relationships
- The decline of genuine spirituality as an ethical force in the culture
- An explosion of information that creates anxiety over one's worth or abilities
- An overreliance on "self" to find the meaning of life[8]

All of these factors can contribute to the adult and teenage dysfunctional behavior that sociologists have charted. Our society is in need of more widespread healing. It seems strange, even a paradox, that some of the same individuals so successful in storing up material gains and striving for power are so often those who have neuroses and psychosomatic complaints. A comedian once asked his audience: "Why is it that only rich people suffer from exhaustion?"

Along these same lines Barbara Shlemon observed that "We are of little value to the Lord when we are self-reliant and dependent upon our own strength."[9] Obviously, there can be a virtue in being self-reliant. It seems, however, that Shlemon is referring to the absence of faith or the failure to acknowledge or call on God's help in reaching out to others. There is no virtue in refusing aid, if we are among those who work with less-than-adequate resources or compassionate motivation at their disposal. By acknowledging our weakness and relying more on God's help, we may find ourselves more spiritually empowered to reach out to those in distress and more energetically address their cries for deliverance from their troubles.

When it comes to healing, there is often a paradox that the more selfless the person, the more effective channel for healing that person can become. Saint Paul may have felt this reality in his question: "Who is weak, and do I not feel weak? . . . If I must boast, I will boast of the things that show my weakness" (2 Corinthians 11:29-30). Paul would have appreciated the truth and humor in the following anonymous witticism: "People who live solely for themselves are eventually corrupted by their own company." Ideally, we need to belong to a community of the unselfish to be assisted in our struggles, to return the favor to those who have helped us, and to test our beliefs and manner of living against a framework larger than ourselves. Obviously such communities could not exist without the virtues of forbearance and mutual forgiveness.

COMMUNITIES OF SUPPORT

Each of us has had special relationships, people in our lives who have been sources of healing for us; in some instances it is the acceptance and forgiveness they have extended to us. They have all come into our lives at various times over a period of many years. Even total strangers have "dropped into" our lives to become sources of divine encounters. In the field of education, for example, there were a number of "saints" previously unknown who appeared seemingly "out of the blue," wonderful people enabling us financially, spiritually, and emotionally. In our shared faith we have recognized these people as having become divine encounters with us at pivotal times of difficulty. However, many more "helpers" along the journey of life have had positive influences in other areas as well. We have all experienced these special, and in some ways, mysterious people who seem to come along at just the opportune moment to provide for a given need. They have become for us the "evidence" that God is always present and tends to our problems. It may not be wholly inaccurate to call these moments "miracles" of divine intervention.

In addition to God's direct and indirect help, we need people who can be our personal source of healing; and we, in turn, must be available for each other's needs within our faith community. The community must, in turn, reach out beyond itself to do its share in promoting healing and reconciliation in our wider world. This healing can begin through something so simple as the forgiveness and intercessory prayer we extend to one another. We are all children of God; in the case of the Christian community, brothers and sisters of Jesus Christ. As Eddie Ensley remarks, "the pain we feel for the world is living testimony to our interconnectedness with it. If we deny this pain, we become like blocked and atrophied neurons, deprived of life's flow . . ."[10] Ensley cautions us not to treat each other like little handcarved puppets, each shape conforming to our own needs and place them in our world. On the other hand, we can let people be themselves and treasure each individual's uniqueness. As the old Hindu proverb has proclaimed: "Help another's boat across, and lo! Thine own has reached the shore."

Franciscan Brother and physician Daniel Sulmasy offers the sound observation that health care providers cannot be effective channels for healing others unless they are in a loving communion with both God and their patients.[11] Strong faith on the part of both the caregiver and the patient are important for a complete healing to take place. This can only be enhanced when both partners have a strong belief in the power of prayer and appreciate each other through a compassionate, forbearing relationship.

INNER HEALING THROUGH FORBEARANCE AND FORGIVENESS

Among the prayers that are offered up for various forms of healing, probably the most underappreciated and difficult-to-deal-with are prayers for the inner healing associated with forgiveness. This is so because, in addition to prayers, psychological counseling and medical help may also be required. For example, in the case of a physical illness (e.g., pneumonia), proper medication and rest can usually bring about restoration of the body to health. But unresolved conflicts may remain with us as deep wounds for years and be difficult to root out and resolve.

Agnes Sanford, well-known teacher of spiritual healing, has long dealt with this problem, writing that her "interest has veered away from the healing of the body and has been guided almost entirely into this deeper area: the healing of the 'soul.' Unless the soul is healed, what use is the wholeness of the body?"[12] She had suffered from depression that eventually was healed by keeping herself open and available to God as well as those who were in ministries of God's outreach to the hurting. "He will send you to the right person, or the right person will come to you at the right time."[13] She notes that in addition to professional help for depression, she found comfort and inner peace by becoming part of nature. Doing gardening enabled her to be one with the earth and its creatures, a fellow member of God's creation. In addition, she recommended doing some joyful, creative project for thirty minutes every day.[14]

Nonetheless, *inner healing* may take weeks, months, or years. This may explain how *physical healing,* largely because of the many advances in medicine, has become a lesser challenge compared to inner emotional and spiritual healing. When dealing with buried heartaches, it takes time to eliminate the defenses of hurtful memories and to erase the old memories. Once this has been accomplished, then new patterns of behavior can be established; this also will take considerable time. Acts of forbearance and mutual forgiveness will be vital to these new paths in which hurtful and vindictive feelings are banished from our memory banks.

Forgiving ourselves our own sins, and forgiving others their "sins" against us, is not an easy feat to accomplish. Unhealed hurts can continue to fester within us, requiring large amounts of energy to keep them under control.[15] As we all experience both large and small hurts, we never cease to depend on God's grace, love, and strength as support for our own inner healing. If we can acknowledge the role we have played in hurting others and being hurt ourselves, we then can better attend to the process of healing ourselves, and with help of the spirit of God within us, we can reach out with compassion to those in the relationship that was the cause of the hurt in the first place. An open wound can be then turned into a barely visible scar. In every relationship we are constantly being hurt in small things or large; the need for forgiveness will never go away. Forgiveness and reconciliation will enable us to live a life of inner peace which is vital to both our healing and spiritual growth. The importance of forgiveness cannot be underestimated. Among the most helpful words we can ever hear when we are hurt are "I'm sorry." The most graced words of relief we can ever give are "I forgive you."

Forgiveness as a healing dynamic also makes good sense given our human condition and sinfulness. We are what we are because of God's constant forgiveness. Knowing this, we can more easily move outward from ourselves to love the Christ in others. To forgive *ourselves* and *others* around us is to help create a community where healing is experienced and angering hurts diminished.

In all efforts to be instruments of a caring God in the ministry of healing, it is important for people to know that, in forgiving others, they are following in the ways of God, our preeminent healer of the wounds that continue to afflict us in our human condition. The pain we assume is real, but so too the reward, as Christians see it, of being so closely linked to Jesus in his ministering to the hurting of all ages. In the words of Jean Vanier:

> Jesus is calling us to speak the truth as he did, to become compassionate and to walk down the ladder into the heart of poverty and pain, both our own and that of others. There we will find the freedom to cherish all the beauty given us, the love, and song, and laughter, and we will then rise up together in a community of forgiveness and celebration knowing what it is to be his Body.[16]

No wonder Vanier found Jesus and God's presence precisely in his own compassionate ministry to overcome the pain of the mentally handicapped through the L'Arche communities of forbearance, forgiveness, and celebration.

Paul's advice to the Christians of Rome is timely in this regard: "As for those who try to make your life a misery, bless them. Don't curse them, bless them. . . . Don't pay back a bad turn by a bad turn to anyone. . . . As far as your responsibility goes, live at peace with everyone" (Romans 12:15-18, J. B. Phillips Translation, New Testament). Commenting on that passage from Romans, Dietrich Bonhoeffer even at the height of Adolf Hitler's preaching hatred of and vengeance against Germany's declared enemies, asked his congregation to take as their example Jesus' prayer of forgiveness of his executioners and his instructions to forgive even one's enemies.

> God gave God's life, God's all, for your enemies; now you, too, give them what you have: bread if they are hungry, water if they are thirsty, aid if they are weak, blessing, compassion, and love for your enemy. . . . When you reject your enemy, you turn the poorest of the poor from your door.[17]

In our present climate in which nursing grudges and "getting even" is acceptable conduct and often lauded in films and pulp fiction, the advice of Paul and Bonhoeffer may seem naive and extreme. Yet the healing described in this book is much more than the physical cure of an illness or even the quasi-miraculous recovery from disease through the skills of modern medical technology. Healing must be holistic, extending to the inner psyche and the very soul of a troubled person. Given the vicissitudes of human life and the ever-changing tides of our personal relationships, including the intimacy of people in love, the attitude of forbearance and forgiveness is a constant energizer for the well-adjusted personality and for relationships of friendship and love to last.

Saint Paul's counsel to his Christians in Galatia is likewise apropos the need of every Christian community for the practice of forbearance: "Carry each other's burdens, and in this way you will fulfill the law of Christ" (Galatians 6:2). That message came after he had associated his new found Christian freedom with the law of love: "The entire law is summed up in a single command: 'love your neighbor as yourself' " (Galatians 5:14). Daniel Day Williams noted in his analysis of the forms of love exemplified by Jesus and Paul, that "mercy, forgiveness and reconciliation are not simply formal ideas of what love ideally is. They are the rendering in human terms of what the love of God is doing in human life."[18] Williams goes on to say that the love of which the scriptures speak does not remove all risk-taking from our lives:

> Love does not end all risk, it accepts every risk which is necessary for its work. Love does not resolve every conflict; it accepts conflict as the arena in which the work of love is to be done . . . Love seeks the reconciliation of every life so that it may share with all the others.[19]

In refusing to love and rejecting efforts at reconciliation, Williams concludes that "we make our hells and we cling to them in our love-lessness."[20]

Despite the positive benefits of the love and a forgiving attitude, some people see such an attitude as out of touch with reality in our culture of violence, domination, and the nagging presence of multiple litigations now cluttering our court systems. Although Americans in large numbers still recite, "forgive us our sins as we forgive those who have sinned against us," in truth many find it difficult to forgive. Psychologist Anna Freud once complained about this harboring of grievances and the psychological problems it presents someone such as her, dedicated to healing the wounded psyche of her patients. Speaking of one of her woman patients, she noted that the woman defied even the best psychoanalysis available.

> I think, frankly, what she really aches to have is forgiveness. She is pursued by her own furies. . . . If she were a bit more religious, if she could get down on her knees and pray, perhaps she would obtain relief. But I doubt she will find that solace. She needs for-giveness—to forgive herself, to be forgiven. In our field, for-giveness is an unknown idea.[21]

Can we, created in God's image, be less than loving and forgiving— as God continues to forgive us our own sins—in relating to others?

Yet, in the Christian tradition and in the stories of Jesus, forgive-ness is not an unknown idea; it is a paramount reality. Of the final words of Jesus recorded by Saint Luke, the most significant in reveal-ing what kind of person he was and what we learn about God from him is his prayer for the forgiveness of his executioners. According to Doris Donnelly, forgiveness is not an easy dynamic in dealing with the pain of physical and emotional violence done to one's well-being. The nonforgiver retains the right to even the score, to stand on princi-ple, to exact "sweet revenge," to punish, to maintain the letter of the law. Sinners must pay the price for their wrongdoing. Our prison sys-tem is itself a coalescence of all those attitudes of and rationale for nonforgiveness.[22] Martin Luther King Jr., for example, called capital punishment—for a majority of Americans the justice system's main deterrent against crime—"society's final assertion that it will not for-give."[23]

Genuine forgiveness, whether of oneself or of others, is itself an essential moment in physical and emotional healing as it is in maintaining healthy relationships. Forgiveness has the immediate effect of removing a major barrier in the process of eliminating stress from one's life when combating the various illnesses that are exacerbated by our personal tensions. To forgive another is to surrender our grudges and desires for retaliation, to pass over our grievances, and not to posture in indignant self-righteousness. Certainly part of the appeal of Jesus to the masses, among whom were the sinners who crowded around him, lay in his never invoking moral superiority. He exuded the holiness of his forgiving Father. He could even speak warmly of the joy to be derived from forgiveness of others, more so than from standing on pedestals of self-righteous refusal to grant pardon for transgressions.

Jesus Christ made it his mission to heal people precisely by forgiving them their sins and considered that more important than any physical healing (Matthew 9:2-8; Mark 2:5-12; Luke 5:20-26). Some scholars maintain that Jesus' forgiveness was the catalytic element in the subsequent miracles of physical restoration. In Luke's Gospel, for instance, Jesus asks his followers not to be judgmental, not to be condemning, and always to forgive (Luke 6:37). Jesus advocated reconciliation even ahead of acts of worship (Matthew 5:23-24). He tied in the forgiveness his followers received to their own willingness to forgive others the sins committed against them. To all he preached what the author of Ephesians asked of the members of that community: "Be kind and compassionate to one another, forgiving each other, just as in Christ God forgave you" (Ephesians 4:32).

The attitude of forgiveness not only lifts the burdens of guilt and deep-seated resentments from our hearts, it also conveys the peace and freedom that are among the most precious gifts in Jesus' legacy to his followers. Forgiveness is the point where justice and mercy meet in the unique encounter that is Jesus' own way, truth and life. Such forgiveness, according to Roger Lovette, Baptist minister in Birmingham, Alabama, is "the centerpiece of all Jesus did." He adds that, in forgiveness, one meets Jesus Christ firsthand. Commenting on the story of Jesus' forgiving the adulterous woman in the face of the self-righteous crowd's desire to punish by stoning her to death, Lovette notes that Jesus sees in the woman the potential she had never experienced. "He reached out in love and care. He took her seriously. He understood also the twisting and winding roads that had led her to that terrible hour." The gift of forgiveness that extended to her and to us "means that we stand up and face the future without the weight of the past."[24]

The prayer ministry with one's patients that we have been advocating is in line with that Gospel encounter. The woman's adultery could symbolize the many sins and guilt feelings that linger as a pounding hangover does, in attempting to begin a new day in good health. Prayer helps alleviate the burdens of guilt that may weigh heavily against the mental equilibrium needed for a complete recovery from an illness. One's frame of mind, one's attitude toward oneself, are adjunct forces in the ministry of healing. Theologian and storyteller Frederick Buechner has said it well:

> When somebody you've wronged forgives you, you're spared the dull and self-diminishing throb of a guilty conscience. When you forgive somebody who has wronged you, you're spared the dismal corrosion of bitterness and wounded pride. For both parties, forgiveness means the freedom again to be at peace inside their own skins and to be glad in each other's presence.[25]

FORGIVENESS IN DIFFICULT CIRCUMSTANCES

In the practical, political sphere, Anglican Bishop Tutu of South Africa, has shown the wider possibilities of forgiveness on a national scale. Bishop Tutu was Chair of South Africa's "Truth and Reconciliation Commission" during the period when it reviewed the many atrocities committed by the South African Government against the native black population. By extending forgiveness to those who admitted their guilt, the commission backed up their resolve with the following statement of policy: "Revenge and retribution merely unleash an inexorable cycle of reprisal provoking counter reprisal."[26] This policy has led to a significant change in attitude, amelioration of the oppression and injustice so widespread previously, and provided a lesson for other nations around the globe to emulate.

Bishop Tutu was interviewed again about whether his feelings on forgiveness had changed following the September 11, 2001, attacks by terrorists on the Twin Towers in New York and on the Pentagon. He reiterated his opinion very forcefully, although he was aware his faith in forgiveness was not in accord with the announced intention of the United States to retaliate militarily for the attacks. Even while he voiced his condemnation of the atrocity, he also declared that, "Forgiveness and reconciliation are not cheap, they are costly." Instead of the planned violent retaliation, he advised that we "choose to recognize the humanity of the perpetrator and thereby give him the possibility of making a new beginning." He added, "it is to hope in the essential goodness of people and have faith in their potential to change."[27]

Tutu summarized his thoughts this way:

> We are in the forgiving business, whether we like it or not. And we can do this only through God's grace. It is ultimately God at work in us to make us to be like God. Yes, it is a tall order, but that is the love that changes the world, that believes the enemy is a friend waiting to be made.[28]

These are words of faith, indeed. These are words of a follower of Jesus Christ who has embraced the Gospel. But they are also words that contradict the vengeful desires of many Americans following the tragedy of September 11, 2001. Seeking out the causes of the hatred of the terrorists, addressing these causes, making an attempt at reconciliation, following Jesus Christ's teachings on peace and forgiveness, were all ideas repudiated by a majority of American citizens. One can only wonder what results could have been achieved had we as a nation listened to Bishop Tutu instead of those who were hawking war as the only solution to acts of terror and citing the national security anxiety that politicians often invoke to justify their militarism.

The emotional uplift that comes from forgiving others the wrongs they have committed against our own person has never been more movingly expressed than in Corrie ten Boom's account of her own difficult struggle to forgive an enemy. She had survived the hell of incarceration in the Ravensbruck concentration camp. Her beloved sister, Betsie, had died there. On her release she began to preach and lecture extensively on the need to forgive one's enemies. After one such lecture she was approached by a man who had been an SS guard in the shower room of the camp. She who had preached forgiveness had now come face to face with one of those responsible for the suffering she had endured at the hands of the Nazis. The man thanked her for her message and the consoling thought that his sins had been washed away by Jesus. Her own thoughts at that moment were of her sister's pain and the horrors of the camp. As the man held out his hand she kept her own hand at her side while her anger and feelings of vengeance boiled up within her. She prayed that the Lord forgive her and, in turn, help her to forgive him. When she still could not raise her hand and was unable to feel any movement of charity toward the man, she prayed again, telling Jesus that she could not forgive but would Jesus give her his forgiveness. At that moment, the burden was lifted.

> As I took his hand a most incredible thing happened. From my shoulder along my arm and through my hand a current seemed to pass from me to him, while into my heart sprang a love for this stranger that almost overwhelmed me. And so I discovered that it is not on our forgiveness any more than our goodness that the world's healing hinges, but on his. When he tells us to love our enemies, he gives, along with the command, the love itself.[29]

That kind of faith in Jesus' words became the force that permitted Corrie ten Boom to love the one who had stood for what in the days of her suffering and grief she had hated.

Not every act of forgiveness is as dramatic as the experience of Corrie ten Boom. Forgiving another the pain he or she has caused is, nonetheless, very difficult. The wound is not on the bodily surface where a physician can examine clinically, and then clean, stitch, and bandage. When a person is deeply hurt to the point of anger and resentment, the wound is festering in one's inner psyche and may take much longer to heal. Christians are, nonetheless, asked by Christ to allow the spirit of forgiveness to work its way to the bottom layer of our spirit where the resentment hangs on. The forgiveness is not automatic; the persons offended are asked to bypass their grief, anger, and lingering antipathy. Forgiveness becomes, then, a power expressed in a difficult-to-do deed. To pardon another is to enable a change in relationship with the person forgiven to take place. Such an undertaking is arduous even for the person of great faith because it brings the forgiver along the path of confronting one's own sinfulness. Henri Nouwen, a priest psychologist and spiritual director conscious of his own shortcomings, observed with uncanny accuracy the progression from awareness of one's own flaws and weakness to the act of forgiveness: "Forgiveness is only real [for the compassionate person] who has discovered the weakness of his friends and the sins of his enemy in his own heart and is willing to call every human being his brother."[30]

Sometimes it takes a modern account of "extreme" forgiveness to stir the imagination of and moral sensitivities of ordinary people. The kindly bishop of *Les Miserables* who forgives Jean Valjean his theft of the bishop's silver and then saves him from a life in prison by pressing on him the gift of the expensive candlesticks he had been accused of stealing, all in the very presence of the gendarmes come to cart him away, succeeds in converting Valjean to a new life of compassion and social justice. To the bishop this seemingly misplaced act of kindness and forgiveness was merely what Jesus would have done. His forgiveness emanated from that peace which he had found in Jesus Christ, which baffles sheer human understanding.

On a more global scale Pope John Paul II emphasized forgiveness in his message for the representatives of the world religions during "The Day of Prayer for Peace in the World" at Assisi, Italy, January 24, 2002. In that message he spoke of the "two pillars" upon which peace rested, namely, "commitment to justice and the readiness to forgive." He went on to remind those assembled at Assisi that forgiveness is crucial to maintaining peace in the world among nations as among people in general "because human justice is subject to frailty and to the pressures of individual and group egoism. Forgiveness alone heals the wounds of the heart and fully restores damaged human relations."[31] In the pope's view just as there can be no true peace without social justice, neither can there be true justice without a willingness of nations and peoples to forgive one another.

Nor can there be the physical, emotional, and mental healing that the sick need unless the attitude of forgiving can become a daily reality in the lives of the caregiver, the patient, and those who are coping with the illness of a loved one. None other than God has given us the example of forbearance and forgiveness in God's relationship with us throughout our lifetimes. The Lord's Prayer is apropos God's own attitude that God's spirit would have us make our own: "Forgive us our sins as we forgive those who have sinned against us."

DISCUSSION QUESTIONS

1. Comment on the assertion that forgiveness has the potential to bring about both spiritual and emotional healing.

2. How can one achieve a change of heart in dealing with feelings of vengeance and getting even? Is it true that negative feelings toward others factor into illness? Explain.
3. Comment on the insight offered by Brother Roger of Taizé.
4. Comment on the story of Emma and her role in spiritual healing.
5. Comment on the claim of Henri Nouwen about self-rejection. How does his statement relate to the need in health care for patients to forgive themselves in order to forgive others in their search for wholeness?
6. The authors claim that when contemporary society encourages isolation, rugged individualism and aggressive self-assertion, this can detract from human relations and attitudes that are important for health care. Do you agree with this? Explain.
7. Describe the societal pressures that can lead to anxiety, lack of forbearance, and ill-health. How can the health care provider counteract these sources of emotional alienation?
8. Comment on the authors' assertion that when it comes to healing, there is often a paradox that the more selfless the person, the more effective the channel for healing that person can become. Does Jesus illustrate this by his example?
9. Describe the impact made by those in our special relationships who at given moments have helped in our healing, whether physical, emotional, or spiritual. Are these people "divine encounters" in our times of difficulty?
10. Comment on the stories of forgiveness and reconciliation in the lives of Jean Vanier, Dietrich Bonhoeffer, Anna Freud, Bishop Tutu, and Corrie ten Boom. Can these stories be related to health care issues?

Chapter 7

Listening from the Heart in Health Care

Whether one's ministry is health care, child care, hospice care, spiritual care, or one spouse caring for the other, listening is an essential virtue. As Oliver Wendell Holmes said, "It is the province of knowledge to speak, and it is the privilege of wisdom to listen."[1] Is not the attractiveness of God to those who suffer related to the simple yet compassionate claim that the Lord hears the cry of the poor (see Psalm 34:6).[2] The prophetic vocation is to listen to the cries of those who have been victimized by life's misfortunes. The charm of Jesus of Nazareth was his ability to listen to the pleas of the underclass of Jewish society that their voices be heard and they be accepted by the one who in their eyes represented none other than a God who cares. As with the rich and the religious leaders, they too were created in God's image and likeness and now they should be welcomed into the Christian community as the hurting brothers and sisters with whom Jesus has made common cause.

In a powerful section of his classic treatise on Christian community, Dietrich Bonhoeffer enjoined on his students in the secret seminary that he was directing under the noses of the Gestapo that they be avid listeners in their respective ministries and that they begin this service in the seminary itself.

> The first service one owes to others in the community, involves listening to them. Just as our love for God begins with listening to God's Word, the beginning of love for other persons is learning to listen to them. God's love for us is shown by the fact that God not only gives us God's Word, but also lends us God's ear. We do God's work for our brothers and sisters when we learn to listen to them.[3]

Is There a God in Health Care?
© 2006 by The Haworth Press, Inc. All rights reserved.
doi:10.1300/5554_07

Bonhoeffer had obviously recognized that the key to the formation of a Christian community close to the ideals and teachings of Jesus Christ depended on the warmth of their personal relationships through the attention one person should extend to the other.

The key to any successful relationships, whether they be personal, community, or even international, requires attentive listening. But equally important for health care providers is to listen to what God is trying to say in their lives. To accomplish this, they must learn to be still and listen to God's word on a daily basis. John Stott coined the term "double listening," to explain listening not only to the voice of God, but also to those voices of people in need coming from a multiplicity of sources across the globe. It involves hearing what the Bible is saying, as well as what ordinary people in today's world are saying.[4]

LISTENING IN THE MODERN WORLD

One might ask which words in the Bible are most compatible with the contributions that medical science and faith-filled caregivers find most helpful. Here the practical wisdom of the Apostle James is to the point. James' wisdom has stretched over 2,000 years and yet is just as pertinent today as in ancient times: "My dear brothers, take note of this: Everyone should be quick to listen, slow to speak and slow to become angry, for man's anger does not bring about the righteous life that God desires" (James 1:19-20). James goes one step beyond listening to the need to make our listening practical for one another in his additional remark: "But be doers of the word, and not merely hearers who deceive themselves" (James 1:22).

Being "quick to listen" is the theme of this chapter. If we speak of listening from the heart to those who cry out to us for relief from their ills both bodily and emotional, we are describing a vital aspect of the vocation of a health care provider. Listening attentively to one's fellow human beings is also an art that can be learned; it is a sign of that humility, respect, and mutual understanding which many great saints had. Bonhoeffer, being an ordained minister himself as well as a seminary director, once made the remark: "They [Ministers] forget that *listening* can be a greater service than speaking."[5] We have already noted that caregivers who sit silent at the bedside of an ill patient can express an inaudible prayer, and become a source of comfort, by just being present. This can be very difficult for physicians to accomplish. First of all, they have been trained to *act,* and not to sit still, at the bedside of a patient, particularly if that patient is terminally ill. Also, they may often have an unrealistic expectation that their patient is not going to die. When the natural event of death occurs, despite all the modern medical advances at their disposal, it can be perceived as a failure on their part.

Then there is the real or imagined thought when confronting a near-death and medically hopeless situation, that doctors must hurry away—excusing themselves with the pretense that "other patients who are also ill now demand their attention." Is this our escape from an uncomfortable and potentially humbling situation? What more can any caregiver do or say to the assembled family? All physicians have struggled with many of these issues, especially during their early years in practice. In those early days, they may have thought they could handle most medical conditions. But they soon recognize their fragility when dealing with dying patients—dying despite all modern scientific medicine could offer. Doctors were trained to aim for a cure, and should the patient die, it often could be interpreted as a failure or the thought that something was missed. Should every recent gas pain have a workup in order to detect whether this is the one in fifty who may have an early tumor? Would a lab test or an X-ray, if done one or two weeks earlier, have made a big difference in the outcome? No pat answers are available, but listening attentively to the history often is the key for making advanced diagnostic tests. The real world dictates that not everyone in the world should have a prophylactic barium enema. Active listening is still the best starting point from a physician's perspective that combines the science of medicine with the practice of one's faith and compassion. It may later prevent a doctor's anguish in dealing with the perennial question when a patient's condition worsens: What if I had only done this or that?

DOCTOR BILL'S PERSONAL REFLECTIONS

At times it may take a medical crisis to effect a dramatic change in the spiritual outlook of either a patient or the physician. The example of Peter comes to mind. Peter was a bright young undergraduate who flunked out of a leading college on the Eastern seaboard due to alcohol addiction. The magnitude of this event both shocked him and sobered him at the same time. He took a year off from school, attended AA meetings and spent time talking to high school and college students about the seriousness of alcohol addiction. He began to listen to what we might label "God's call" moving him to enter another undergraduate institution, and from there to a seminary, where he happily "graduated" with high honors. He is now a well-respected priest. We have noted a number of stories such as his, where a strong setback to an individual resulted in a renewed and energetic spiritual journey. As with so many stories, it may take a jolt to belatedly open the door for God to enter and for us to *listen* for his guidance.

Listening for such divine guidance is not always easy. In fact, it often takes considerable patience to be able to listen to the woes of another. The following story of one of my patients may illustrate what a health caregiver may have to endure in extending compassionate listening to another. A middle-aged woman, accompanied by her husband, arrived one day for an initial office visit. She appeared distraught, as did her husband. She carried a paper bag filled with bottles of medications. This could not help but catch my eye. Through the grace of God and the power of the Spirit, I listened for almost a solid hour without interrupting, as she related a veritable litany of complaints. This encompassed an extended "laundry list" of problems, enough to fill a major textbook of medicine. With fine detail, she covered every item. She then turned to me and said, "No one has let me describe all my symptoms before!" Little did she know that all the time I was praying for the gift of endurance in the midst of my growing fatigue at her protracted tale of woe. But my prayers were answered; I was enabled to listen attentively and to get a clearer picture of the source of her troubles. The extra bonus for both of us was that the lady had become more trusting. Over time she was willing to gradually eliminate the bulk of her medications as the former contents of her paper bag were lessened week by week. Eventually most of her initial symptoms had been alleviated; she had more energy, and reported that she "did not feel drugged anymore." As an added bonus, her husband greatly appreciated the fact that the reduced prescriptions meant an equally important drop in the cost of her medication.

This was a success that would not have been possible without the Spirit's help at the initial visit. Along with my reassurances, a modest exercise program, and the elimination of most of her pills, a major victory had been won! Something can be gleaned from the story of a wise old owl: Wise old owl lived in an oak; The more he saw the less he spoke; The less he spoke the more he heard: Why can't we all be like that bird? (Edward Hersey Richards).

Often enough, an impediment to being a good listener to others, even in their complaints, is making judgments based upon preconceived attitudes, stereotypes, and judgments. While living in the Spirit, we must pray for help in ridding ourselves of these premature judgments. My encounter with George made me realize my own weakness in this regard. I had rushed to a false conclusion about him. George is a very well-known hospital worker who taught me a salutary lesson in both listening to and judging people. We were in line waiting to pay the cashier in the hospital cafeteria a few years ago, and to my surprise and disdain, I overheard George screaming at the cashier for some reason unknown to me. The cashier was well liked by all in the hospital family. The altercation initiated by George both puzzled and annoyed me greatly. Of course, I then labeled George in my mind as an unreasonable person and someone I could not possibly deal with. After about two years of avoiding each other, one day we found ourselves alone in the elevator. I then looked at George and asked how things were going for him, and the surprising response was one of the broadest of grins that I have ever seen. He became alive to me, and, I guess, I to him.

From that moment on, I realized he might not be such a bad person after all. He might even be likable! I noted for the first time the pins indicating years of hospital service on his jacket. It then occurred to me that he must have done at least a few things well. It was not long before we became good friends. Today, whenever I enter the front door of the hospital or am working on one of the hospital floors, I frequently will hear a voice from a long distance down a corridor shouting, "Hi, Doc!" It is George waving and smiling, his gold teeth shining in the daylight. He loves to watch local college basketball. Guess what? He wears my Princeton orange and black suspenders to every home game! The biblical reminder is very apropos our tendency to rush to judgment of others: "Do not judge, or you too will be judged" (Matthew 7:1).

THEOLOGIAN GEFF'S
PERSONAL REFLECTIONS

At times, actively listening to God and living in his presence is a community event. Most people need the support of a community of believers to help them on their way to physical as well as spiritual health. The community gives needed spiritual and emotional support, and also serves to keep our spiritual journey on course. Otherwise unknowingly, we may wander off in a different direction becoming our own Holy Spirit and our own solitary church. The listening community serves as a resource for affirmation as well as correction in the direction of one's spirituality. Bonhoeffer's own spiritual classic study of Christian community reinforces the importance of this community connection. At the same time, he cautions the community to remember that the ministry of listening to one another will be the gauge of just how Christian the community may be despite its claims to be following Jesus Christ. His words are uncompromising on this virtue.

> But Christians who can no longer listen to one another will soon no longer be listening to God either; they will always be talking even in the presence of God. The death of the spiritual life starts here, and in the end there is nothing left but empty spiritual chatter and clerical condescension which chokes on pious words. Those who cannot listen for a long time and patiently will always be talking past others, and finally no longer will even notice it. Those who think their time is too precious to spend listening will never really have time for God and others, but only for themselves and for their own words and plans.[6]

These are apt words for health caregivers and religious people alike.

Bonhoeffer connects this kind of listening to the ability to practice silence and enjoy moments of solitude in prayer. A whole section of his book on community is devoted to "The Day Alone." Silence is not exactly considered a virtue in this noisy age in which tastes in music and film tend to favor the loud, the explosive, and the shouting of opinions one to another. Is this a new phenomenon? Paul Tournier, a Swiss internist, wrote a few decades ago that we humans have not changed very much over time.

Modern people lack silence. They no longer lead their own lives; they are dragged along by events. It's a race against the clock. If your life is chock-full already, there won't be room for anything else; even God can't stuff anything else in.[7]

Tournier, a spiritually sensitive physician, has become a role model for caregivers. He strongly believes that doctors must be freed from their scientific prisons, and that medicine is more than science; it is about the humanity of people. To have a valid spiritual connection, physicians must cast off the notion that they know more than the patient. The ability for their patients to talk honestly about their inner concerns is related to physicians' being able to open their own hearts and to be available to them. We are to look upon the patient as a whole person rather than considering him or her a "case" or a scientific challenge. Health caregivers have found that one of the great joys in medicine is developing a special trust between the caregiver and the person who has come for help.

This blending of science and faith is well described by Tournier: "To bear witness to my own faith is to awaken in him (or her) those spiritual forces which give structure, life, and unity to him (or her) as a person."[8] According to Tournier, a certain blend of warmth and commitment supports the suffering patient; enabling doctors and others involved in health care to see themselves confronting the illness as well as aiding the patient in the healing process.

Those whose listening is directly connected to the sense of the presence of God, know that it is in the quietness of the soul that one obtains the inner peace necessary to be a good health care provider. The Hebrew scriptures reinforce the importance of listening to God as he speaks to those who can turn their hearts to the divine presence: "Let me hear what he the Lord will speak, for he will speak peace to his people, to his faithful, to those who turn to him in their hearts" (Psalm 85:8).

Frederick Buechner offers sentiments close to this exhortatory prayer of the Psalmist. In his book, *The Sacred Journey,* he refuses to endorse the distinction between chance happenings in our lives and what seems to happen because of God's intervention. But he insists at the same time that there is no chance occurrence in which God does not speak.

He speaks, I believe, and the words he speaks are incarnate in the flesh and blood of our selves and of our own footsore and sacred journeys. We cannot live our lives constantly looking back, listening back, lest we be turned to pillars of longing and regret, but to live without listening at all is to live deaf to the fullness of the music. . . . [God] says he has been with us since each of our journeys began. Listen for him. Listen to the sweet and bitter airs of your present and your past for the sound of him.[9]

Buechner's advice is timely for those who complain that they experience the seeming absence of God more often than any feeling that God is present. Listening to God, he seems to say, is akin to listening to ourselves and to those who may represent for us the voice of God in happenings, some planned, such as a powerful liturgy, some happenstance or even crisis driven where chaos appears to gnaw at the bones of our well-being.

The Reverend William Tully of St. Bartholomew's Church in New York City has himself experienced just how crucial this act of listening can be even when people are caught up in the daily, often humdrum activities of daily living. "*Listen* to your life," he advised in a memorable sermon:

Take time to get below its every day details, and you will begin to hear the voice of God. That is how the spirit of God works. Very few people are mystics, or have mountaintop experiences, but all have this trivia and this routine, and we miss its true meaning.[10]

What Tully appears to be saying is that God walks with us amid all our bother with and fussiness about the nitty details of our daily schedule. Alhough we may see these many details—we risk missing God's presence.

The essence of good listening is always compassion for the other person. At times this may entail entering into the feelings and attitudes of the other while letting go of any preoccupation that we may have with ourselves. Bishop Thomas Shaw, a prominent Anglican bishop from Massachusetts, has shared an insight into these attitudes that he received while driving his car. He is unique among bishops in that he prefers to live as a monk in a monastery instead of in a typical bishop's residence. His story in summary form tells of an unexpected epiphany that took place while giving a ride to a stranger. One day, upon leaving a church service in a nearby town and about to drive off, a stranger asked for a ride back to his home. He knew the bishop and he lived in Cambridge. What the stranger did not know was that Bishop Shaw was really going to the airport and a drive to Cambridge was out of his way. Yet, in a burst of generosity and compassion, he said yes to the stranger anyway.

During the ride, he learned what a good person the stranger was as he listened to him unravel the story of his life and of the spiritual moments that had affected his faith so strongly. That hour's drive out of his way blessed Shaw's life as it dawned upon him that he had been becoming cynical in his own journey and that this stranger, who was not in any church ministry, was in his own way truly a "man of God." In listening to this stranger, Shaw realized that he had become too busy, too much living in the future and the past, and not as alert to the presence and word of God in his present busyness. Nor was he as concerned as this stranger to the presence of God in others. He concluded that we often do not live fully in the moment; nor do we listen to the way God speaks to us through those who enter our lives in ordinary as well as in the unpredictable intrusions into our everyday existence. It dawned on him that there is a need to be alert to God's presence and voice in the *now* moments. He was even missing the lessons he had learned in the monastery. Contemplation is, above all, living with God in the *now* moment by quiet awareness of God's presence. In many of his sermons and lectures, Shaw recounts that when he travels by air from Boston, as the plane flies over his monastery, he begins to leave all his cares behind. By the time the plane is above the clouds, there is "openness"—no earthly distractions, leaving an opening for God to speak. Shaw cites this as an example of being free—to receive the gift of God's undivided presence and attention. For him this has always been a healing moment.

When not traveling, Bishop Shaw spends time in the morning employing the "breathing prayer." As he breathes in, he repeats, "Come, Holy Spirit," and exhales all of his concerns. This practice has helped many people over the centuries. He conceives of his spiritual journey as one devoted to uncovering layer after layer of attachments to people, places, or things, similar to peeling an onion. He lets these go in order to be closer to God who is free from all petty attachments.

Bishop Shaw is convinced that, since we are made in the image of God, we can adopt a more God-like attitude toward the trivialities of life. Being detached gives freedom to the person of prayer. By contemplation, he says, the worries of the world can be replaced by an awareness of God and the gift of God's own word. Over time, and in communion with the many saints who have listened to God's word, one can experience God's healing presence in all things.[11]

SOME PRACTICAL REFLECTIONS

Realistically, not everyone is a good listener, although the art of listening can be acquired. Here are some practical suggestions. These were developed through my personal experience in working with groups to develop a better ability to hear those who may depend on our attentive listening in order for us to provide for their health care needs.

- A listener must take the time even when it is not convenient.
- Personal issues must be placed aside during this time.
- Remain calm even when the sick person is demanding, manipulative, or demonstrates a spectrum of negative characteristics.
- Despite any negative characteristics, the upset person must be seen as a fellow human being—a child of God—and therefore must be approached with a sense of love.
- Once we are committed as a helper or companion, we must be there when needed, and this may spread out over a lengthy period of time.
- In the case of the dying patient or one suffering from a chronic illness, sharing the journey may require extra amounts of serenity and endurance.
- The compassionate listener companion soon learns the value of doing just little things such as getting a glass of water, fluffing the pillows, lifting the shades, arranging cards or flowers, etc.
- Being present may be more consoling for the ill person than being presented with a number of medications for minor complaints.
- Professional caregivers expect to be in control, and in the case of hospice or terminally ill patients, the roles are best reversed.

- At times, the caregiver may find that the patient has the same illness he or she has and even admire the courage and grace that the patient demonstrates. The caregiver is, therefore, "not alone" in bearing the same diagnosis. It is okay to allow the patient to be in control while the doctor or caregiver *listens.*

We hasten to add this anonymous bit of sound advice: "Do not walk behind me. I may not lead. Do not walk in front of me. I may not follow. Just walk beside me and be my friend" (Anonymous).

The listener who becomes a caring friend can be a catalyst for spiritual growth. By knowing the individual's whole story, we can point out the many gifts that often emanate from his or her illness, such as compassion, increased openness, humility, and the power of healing prayer. The helper can experience firsthand love in action and how this can ease one's suffering.

In addition to the previous advice on how to become a good listener, there are also practical suggestions for those involved in the scientific practice of medicine and these qualities involve active listening conscious of one's healing ministry.

- Do not anticipate what the patient may want to say, instead, just be present to the individual. Listen! Surprising things may happen.
- At the start, the doctor with the aid of attentive listening may find that what was thought to be an easy diagnosis was not the correct one after all, and with further listening, a different cause altogether became more likely.
- The act of being present and thereby allowing the patient to express his or her symptoms is itself therapeutic.
- Listening to all the details of a person's problems instills a degree of trust in the doctor so that further recommendations or tests that may be suggested become more acceptable and reasonable to the patient.

In our view, then, the core of a successful medical practice revolves around listening attentively and communicating to all who have a role in the patient's welfare. This may require frequent updates, even many times a day, especially for those who are critically ill. The patient, family, friends, nurses, house staff, paramedical people, and all involved must be kept informed.

PATIENTS NEED SOMEONE TO LISTEN TO THEM:
DOCTOR BILL'S EXPERIENCE

One Sunday afternoon I visited a patient of mine. It was really a so-cial visit, as she was on the surgical floor recovering from abdominal surgery. She mentioned how pleased she was that her pastor paid her a call in the hospital an hour earlier. The pastor correctly obtained a brief resumé of her status following the surgery. After greeting her, he said a prayer for her rapid recovery and then said good-bye and left her room. Although she greatly appreciated the call, she said, "I wished he had asked me what we should pray about. Then I would have mentioned to him that what bothered me most was not the pain from the operation, but, instead, it was the pain in my heart due to my daughter's drug addiction. I needed his prayers for this."

It was a lesson for all of us that, as good an idea it is to visit the sick, it is essential to first listen to the story and then be in a better position to ask the question, "Are there any deep concerns that we can pray for?" The good deed was somewhat attenuated by the fact that the clergyperson, although he correctly knew the diagnosis, having spo-ken to the surgical nurse beforehand, had come to the conclusion that her recent surgery was her major concern—not realizing her daugh-ter's problems should have taken precedence.

How many times have we all tried to put the correct word in the mouth of a person afflicted with a problem of stuttering? It requires patience as we wait for the individual to express the proper word. One of my patients remarked to me not too long ago, "I get so damn mad when the person I'm talking to tries to put the word I'm struggling to pronounce in my mouth for me . . . especially when it's the wrong one!"

The same need for heartfelt listening occurs when communicat-ing with patients who have trouble speaking following a stroke or laryngectomy (surgery on the voice box), and those who cannot speak at all, having been placed on a ventilator. A number of creative ways can be used to communicate with these individuals; and a pro-fessional caregiver can suggest some of them for the visitor. Again, patience and an attentive ear are essential in health care. A dear el-derly patient of mine was in the ICU (intensive care unit) and unable to communicate with his wife because he required a ventilator to sus-tain his breathing. He was suffering from the end stages of congestive heart failure, having sustained a number of heart attacks in recent years. He and his spouse were unable to say their "good-byes" vocally. However, it was their wish that he be removed from the respirator in order to accomplish this last act of love and communication. We were fully aware that this would likely hasten his demise. The respirator was removed. They could hold hands and be a silent but eloquent presence to each other as a peaceful death ensued soon afterward. His wife thanked me for allowing those last precious moments to be shared between them.

Equally important is to listen to one's own body. A fifty-two-year-old professor came to the office with the complaint of losing his speech and noting transient weakness in his right leg and arm. He admitted that the "spells" were increasing in frequency, but, he thought they were not serious since, as he said, "they only lasted for a minute or two." It took weeks of persuasion by me and a consulting neurosurgeon for him to allow us to accomplish the necessary tests which ultimately led to the diagnosis of a leaking brain aneurysm. The surgery went well, and I felt relieved after hearing this from the surgeon in the afternoon. But by nightfall, the surgeon reported that the professor had lost his speech and the use of his right arm and leg, just what we hoped surgery would prevent! That night I prayed for the professor and the following morning I continued to pray for him. With great anxiety I entered the ICU where the patient was being observed. You can imagine my relief when I was greeted by the professor as he said, "Hi, Bill!" and simultaneously he raised his right hand and waved! The paralysis had gone and his speech had returned. I breathed a deep sigh of gratitude. He would be cured and return to teaching once more! The professor had listened to his body, tried to deny the symptoms, and only with strenuous efforts on the part of several caregivers, did he act upon it. Had he not, today he would likely be dead or disabled for life.

Listening may also encompass what was *not* said. A thought-provoking example of how this may occur was recounted in one of Anthony de Mello's inimitable parables of wisdom: When a man whose marriage was in trouble sought his advice, the Master said, "You must listen to your wife." The man took this advice to heart and returned after a month to say that he learned to listen to every word his wife was saying. Said the Master with a smile, "Now go home and listen to every word she isn't saying."[12]

As with so many of de Mello's stories and Sherlock Holmes's famous case of the dog who did not bark, this one contains a paradox. How can one listen to what is not spoken? Sometimes emotions such as anger, sorrow, confusion, fear, even joy can be seen clearly on the countenance of a loved one or, conversely, on the face of someone who is neither loved nor friendly. It certainly often occurs when a physician examines a taciturn patient or a patient who just will not cooperate in answering questions. It can be a problem in nearly every aspect of health care and in human relationships. In short, de Mello is touching on another important aspect of listening, that of establishing an empathetic relationship with those for whom we care to the point of being able to sense what they may be saying with their bodily language or with the unvoiced emotions that indicate trouble or happiness.

SUMMARY REFLECTIONS

The joy of the healer who listens to and helps someone in need is the joy of having gifted that person with love and caring attention. In tending to the health problems of those who suffer from various illnesses it is encouraging to know that health care providers have the graced potential to become God's channels of healing and inner peace. Amazing things can happen when needy individuals open up their hearts to another person. Compassionate listeners are crucial to the healing process—they bring light and encouragement to a world too often darkened by today's violence and suffering and to hearts whose complaint may be that nobody listens to them and that therefore no one cares about them.

Gerald Kamens, a volunteer for hospice care in Virginia, looks on his vocation of the past twenty-five years, caring for those in the last stages of their lives, as primarily that of heartfelt listening. Kamens is unique in that he makes bereavement calls. He phones survivors to offer consolation in their emotional pain and fears. He does not give advice. As he puts it, "I am supposed to listen, one hopes with care, compassion, and intelligence, to those thoughts and fears the bereaved person may be reluctant to share with most others; about anger, doubts and 'if onlys.' " By just listening, not so much talking, he assists those grieving to keep in their hearts the memories of their loved ones with all their joys as well as their moments of sadness.

What is the force that keeps him in this calling so filled with the experience of death and grief? His life continues to be focused on providing palliative care for those who are no longer able to be cured by the best medical interventions. His patients will die. He can only offer the comfort of the occasional word tempered by his obvious love for those who are going to that "better place" after their death. He says that he still does hospice care because he has so much "to learn from those whose grief and concerns I try to assuage. More to appreciate in those sudden and fleeting communions that sometimes come to pass between us. I doubt I will ever know why for certain. But I plan to keep on listening." At that apex moment between life and death he has learned much about the meaning of life from those who have opened "a part of their soul" to him.[13]

What Kamens does as his response to the call of the Lord is supported by the scriptures which abound in examples of the blessings to be found in listening to those who cry out for compassion and healing. For many, listening to others can provide a time and patience-consuming challenge. We have a constant urge to speak or to actually do something for one another. Whether it is listening to God, our fellow human beings, our bodies, or even to the sounds of nature itself, we are enhancing our humanity and contributing in our own way to the betterment of a hurting society. The laudatory commendations of successful teachers nearly always contain a clause that the teacher was available to the students and could listen respectfully to their problems and offer them the help they need. How many medical malpractice lawsuits could be avoided if doctors were to listen with the same attentiveness that we have advocated?

DISCUSSION QUESTIONS

1. Can we paraphrase Bonhoeffer's statement to read: "The first service health care providers owe their patients involves listening to them."
2. Comment on the assertion that God's love for us is shown by the fact that God not only gives us God's word, but also lends us God's ear.
3. Discuss the implications for health of the declaration by the Apostle James: "You must understand this, my beloved: let ev-

eryone be quick to listen, slow to speak, slow to anger, for your anger does not produce God's righteousness" (James 1:19-20).

4. Is there any truth in the assertion that listening can be a greater service than speaking in health care? Explain.
5. What lessons can we take from the case of Peter, a recovered alcoholic?
6. How can listening to others help health care providers as well as people in general avoid prejudgments and false judgments about those with whom they come in contact?
7. Comment on Bonhoeffer's assertion on listenting.
8. What application to our society can we make of Paul Tournier's statement on p. 145. How can our noisy age contribute to a failure to listen to one another?
9. Comment on Frederick Buechner's declaration on listening. How do we listen to God?
10. Discuss the practical suggestions for good listening between health care providers and their patients. Can we apply this to hospice care as Gerald Kamens does? Explain.

Chapter 8

Social Responsibility, Compassion, and Spirituality at the National and International Level

The United States has been called a "sick society." Such a designation, whether accurate or inaccurate, usually follows headline snatching acts of random violence, the malicious indiscriminate taking of human life, evidence of widespread homelessness, destitution, and racial discrimination, the revelation of massive business corruption leading to the impoverishment of the common people, and the pervasive drug culture that has stymied police efforts to bring it under control. The list could go on. In each instance, we get a glance at the less-than-attractive side of American history. Those involved in various peace movements complain that American militarism, jingoism, and imperialistic arrogance are symptoms of a deeply embedded neurosis that endangers the health and spiritual faith of millions. For the promoters of peace with justice in our country, Martin Luther King Jr.'s sobering assessment of the problem of United States militarism is worth remembering: "A nation that continues year after year to spend more money on military defense than on programs of social uplift is approaching spiritual death."[1]

Just as a physician has to be completely honest in assessing illnesses in individuals and their causes, so too honesty compels that the illnesses of a nation be likewise diagnosed and their causes properly addressed. It seems ludicrous to speak of spirituality and the health care ministry if national and international policies are such that millions are made to suffer needlessly. The churches and people of faith, whose spirituality should inspire changes in these policies to the point of instigating effective action for justice, appear to be either silent or quite impotent in their response. This is an issue that intersects

Is There a God in Health Care?
© 2006 by The Haworth Press, Inc. All rights reserved.
doi:10.1300/5554_08

both health care and spirituality. In this chapter we will discuss the spirituality and health care that are needed on a national and international level, where the forms of suffering can be more massive than the individual cases we have previously examined. Too often the government treats only the side effects of the health troubles of those most affected by its policies without examining in any serious way the core reason for the problems in the first place. This issue was expressed in simplistic yet compelling terms by Archbishop Dom Helder Camara, who was famous for his defense of the poor in his native Brazil, even going so far as to sell off his archbishop's mansion and move in with the poor in Recife. "Why is it," he asked, "when I give to the poor, they call me a saint? When I ask why the poor have no food, they call me a communist."[2]

Evidence of "sickness" at the national and international level should come as no surprise. The suffering endured through wars and disease on such an unbelievably massive scale points out the horrors of international conflicts and widespread oppression that began in individual countries and regions. The ruthless leaders behind those conflicts have been identified. They were permitted to plot their repressive policies in secret and then to set their evil in motion through tactics of terror and physical coercion against a weakened, scattered opposition. For example, after he had killed millions of his own citizens in the 1930s, Joseph Stalin was quoted as having remarked: "One human death is a tragedy; a million is a statistic."[3] Today in the United States we call such statistics of civilian war dead "collateral damage."[4]

Examining the illnesses of this nation, and the unchecked diseases both national and international, will certainly involve statistics of neglect and examples of governmental policies that hurt ordinary citizens. Yet the grist of this chapter is to assess how these policies affect health care and how such policies call for a critique and confrontation energized by one's spiritual faith. Our questions are double: What can be done to alleviate the suffering due to national and international policies and the ideologies behind them? What role do faith and spirituality play in attempts to heal the wounds caused by those who seem, through their cruel political policies, to have conspired to make life miserable for so many of their vulnerable citizens? These explorations will take us into the areas of poverty and human destitution, ecology and environmental health, corporate greed and its impact on health care, and violence at home together with militarism abroad with their destructive consequences for the nation and the world. The issues we raise are related to justice, compassion, and the active pursuit of peace, all connected intersections with the medical care that, in spiritual terms, is placed within the broader spectrum of divine providence acting through those in the healing professions, peace movements, and agencies for social justice.

POVERTY, FAITH, AND THE MISSION TO ALLEVIATE SUFFERING

Providing health care to all the citizens of a country would appear to be a mandate for any civilized country. Yet in the United States universal health care, common in most civilized countries, has not yet become the law of the land. The fact that over 44 million citizens have no medical insurance and often are not able to receive standard medical services is a standing contradiction of the political boast that the United States has the best medical system in the world. This is true enough if one measures medical care by the presence of advanced diagnostic and interventionist technology in the United States. But it is not enough of the truth, if we look at the nation's ineffective safety net which fails to adequately help many of the poor. This problem is compounded by the lingering statistics of disease and death among the nation's underclass who are bereft of proper medical coverage and unable in many cases to pay for their prescriptions.

The poverty of the overwhelming masses of people in the world is a reality that religious leaders and health care providers have attempted to address with ever-increasing frustration. Part of the problem with those who hold the levers of power in areas where destitution, hunger, and disease are daily realities is the inability of political leaders to understand what the poor have to face. These same politicians exhibit an unwillingness to face the issues that doctors have in establishing continuity of care faced, as they are, with the fragmentation of relationships through HMOs' tight-fisted management of rising costs and, at times, their unwarranted intrusions into standard medical practice.

The German spiritual leader of the resistance movement against Nazism, Dietrich Bonhoeffer, urged his fellow conspirators to see evil through the eyes of the victims:

> There remains an experience of incomparable value. We have for once learned to see the great events of world history from below, from the perspective of the outcast, the suspects, the maltreated, the powerless, the oppressed, the reviled—in short, from the perspective of those who suffer.[5]

He was referring to the Jews and those lingering in death camps throughout Germany and the occupied countries. One can only wonder how a bill for universal health insurance would fare in the Congress of the United States if the representatives and senators could learn to see the problem from the perspective of the uninsured and underinsured, seemingly victimized by a strange indifference to their plight in the halls of Congress.

To their credit, some American politicians have become spokespersons for the poor and have proposed legislation to alleviate their condition or to provide the necessities of life, such as Medicare and food stamps. But politicians such as the late Paul Wellstone have been a rarity in recent times in their espousal of the causes advanced by those mired in less than humane living conditions. For the most part, it is difficult for comfortable legislators or executives to understand the raw experiences of those living in pockets of destitution on the underside of urban America. Bonhoeffer's words were a challenge to his fellow conspirators to see the world of concentration camps and a world at war through the eyes of the victims.

Bonhoeffer's exhortations are also a reminder that we as a nation should try to understand poverty from the perspective of the marginalized people. They may not be able to get or hold a job and, therefore, cannot boast of prosperity. The poor and the powerless have come to know with increasing indignation and bitterness that their needs and rights have been restricted by the political leaders who have neither class nor religious links to them and little appreciation of what it means to live in the grinding poverty of the crime-infested ghettos of North America. How many politicians have ever experienced the hunger of poor people or gone without adequate medical coverage?

The problem of poverty with its adverse effect on health care is compounded by crass ignorance of what poverty really does to people. If Congress were truly serious about lifting people out of their dependency on welfare, it would go far beyond time limits on benefits to the unemployed and seemingly unemployable. It would publicly admit in all honesty that to end welfare dependency will cost far more in the short term. It would involve providing a job to any welfare recipient who continues to be unable to find work. That would cost billions of dollars, money that the United States Congress has diverted to increasing the manufacture of instruments of mass destruction. Instead of seriously examining the plight of the millions of Americans trapped in seemingly inescapable poverty, including some 14 million who subsist on Aid to Families with Dependent Children (AFDC)[6] (The United States government now calls this Temporary Assistance to Needy Families [TANF]), some members of the House of Representatives believe in the dogma that government lavishes too much on poor people, especially those on welfare. An editorial in the *Wall Street Journal* complained that poor people were not paying their share of taxes. The editorial complained that, compared to the percentage of taxes paid by the rich, the poor were not paying an equal percentage. The editor called those "profiting" from this disparity "lucky duckies"![7] The replies to that editorial pointed out just how cold-hearted were his remarks and how oblivious the writer must have been to the unpleasant prospect of living on $12,000 per year.

Advocates for the poor are asking the difficult questions about why Congress intends to cut funding for social projects and still bestow tax breaks on the wealthiest citizens. Across the nation, states have been affected by these measures to the point of being forced to save money by draconian measures such as releasing inmates from their prisons and making drastic cutting of funds for social programs and education. This has resulted in a growing concentration of poverty in inner-city neighborhoods. What this does to the health of those affected by this cycle should be obvious.

First, except for those receiving the slim coverage of Medicaid, who, in turn, complain of the inadequate health care doled out to them, a good number of those at this level of economic hardship cannot afford preventive health maintenance or even the medicines needed to cope with their illnesses. By any canons of distributive justice this constitutes an ethically challenged system. Measured against the moral teachings of the Torah and of Jesus Christ, it is an infidelity to a core mandate of the Judeo-Christian religious tradition. In the United States today, a full 18 percent of the nonelderly population with severe medical problems lack any health insurance at all. Many elderly citizens are unwelcome clients for the HMOs.[8] That does not include those whose insurance is insufficient for their needs or who are only occasionally insured.

The United States is, in fact, the only industrialized nation in the Western world without universal health coverage. Many of the uninsured have employment but with companies that offer no health insurance benefits. Many small businesses claim they can no longer afford medical coverage. By any moral calculus, this is a less-than-adequate condition that cries out for redress. The financing of health care for all the underinsured, as it now stands, is regressive. Dr. Uwe Reinhardt, professor of political economy and professor of economics and public affairs at Princeton university, is considered an authority in health care delivery. He sees no proof that a market-driven health care system is better than a government-driven one; Medicare, with some faults, is still a better choice over a private insurance plan. We are heading for a four-tier system of care. The uninsured will get emergency care, but no ongoing care for chronic illnesses. Medicaid patients will likely receive some partially rationed care. Those in the upper and middle income level will afford enhanced Medicare or an expanded health plan. Individuals in the top 5 to 10 percent income level can receive virtually undamaged care without any rationing. "Beware Orwellian 'efficiency,' " Reinhardt cautions. *Efficiency* properly used is powerful and good; misused it is Orwellian in its nature.[9]

In 2000, there were over 1,300 health insurance plans, but companies may not be licensed in all jurisdictions, as is the case in the successful mandate for Medicare.[10] In the Princeton Medical Center alone there were thirty different HMO plans. Each plan had its own fee schedule, reasons for denial of care, and delayed payment which, for some plans, meant a delay of a year or more. HMOs going bankrupt or merging with other plans have resulted in the loss of doctor-patient relationships. In one recorded instance in Princeton, the comptroller of an institution ordered a new HMO plan for budgetary reasons. The outcome thus destroyed twenty-five years of medical care by mandating a transfer of insurance provider to a new physician and assignment to another hospital. The needless expense and time spent in seeing personally the family doctor for a referral to an HMO-chosen specialist, who might not be as highly qualified as the one the family doctor would have chosen, compounds the problem for most physicians. Certain allowable "fees" are approved by Medicare, according to the diagnosis, but Medicare will "pay" only a percentage of the allowed "fee" in every case. Meantime, office practice overhead expenses continue to rise. Adding to the aggravation faced by health caregivers is the documented fact that the salaries paid to the CEOs (chief executive officers) of HMOs are in the many millions while, at the same time, premiums and costs to physicians and patients skyrocket, and payment to hospitals, physicians, and other caregivers are lowered. Many physicians in private practice desire a medical system where universal coverage and a single payer operate and a necessary degree of compassionate autonomy is restored to the family doctor.

If we invoke the mandates of caring for the sick and injured that are found in the Jewish Torah, the Christian Gospel, and the Islamic Quran, then prophetic outrage at the inequity of our health care system may be called for. In most religious traditions compassion for the poor, the homeless, those suffering from various forms of chronic or acute illness is seen as the sign of one's faith. Physicians who pray with and for their patients have become even more alert to this aspect of their healing ministry.

Few spiritual writers have described the plight of the have-nots of American society with greater passion than Jean Vanier, whose mission is centered on the emotionally and physically distressed. He writes,

> The poor can be the economically poor, who are hungry, homeless and out of work, or the rejected ones—those put aside because of their infirmities and handicaps, their apparent uselessness. They are longing to be accepted and loved, longing for meaning and a healing relationship. The poor are those caught up in sin, yet craving also to be liberated from it. The poor are also any of us who are sad and alone, feeling guilty and unloved. The poor know their own emptiness. They do not hide from it. They long for a savior who will heal their hearts and bring them peace.[11]

The spirituality of a Jean Vanier is needed in our world today. We as health caregivers must, in addition to our daily ministry, pray and work for an increased sensitivity to global injustice and poverty. Our outreach is not limited to our own domestic needs alone. A vital part of our ministry is to encourage the prosperous West to reach out with compassion rather than self-interest to those communities and nations crying out for help. The prophet Jeremiah speaks of the ubiquitous need for hope in these stirring words: "Surely I know the plans I have for you, says the Lord, plans for your welfare and not for harm, to give you a future with hope" (Jeremiah 29:11). The gap between the "haves and have-nots" has steadily increased over the past couple of decades. The United States seems to have largely downplayed the many needs of the Third World in all fields of health, water, food, housing, sanitation, air quality, and building up of infrastructures of poor nations. "The Western standard of living cannot be universalized. It can only be sustained at the expense of people in the 'Third World,' at the expense of coming generations, and the expense of the earth," according to Jurgen Moltmann.[12] More than 2 billion people around the world suffer from Chronic mineral and vitamin deficiencies. Six million children worldwide under the age of five die each year as a result of malnutrition.[13]

Our country has, instead, devoted large sums of money to further isolate itself from the problems of underdeveloped, needy nations. We have become known for being arrogant, rich, and aggressive in directions that are supposedly in our own interests at the cost of those who have none of the above. The United States represents 5 percent of the world's population yet consumes 25 percent of the world's energy.[14] Ironically, while we are instituting programs to cut down on the problem of obesity, over a billion people in the world go to bed hungry every night. According to the American Heart Association, obesity increases risk of cardiovascular disease by its adverse effects on blood lipids, and is a major risk factor for a heart attack.[15] About two-thirds of American adults twenty years of age or older are overweight and one-third of these are obese. Is there any wonder that, because of our "conspicuous consumption," we are now disliked by several nations including some of our former allies? Of the billions of dollars to be spent on missile defense, has anyone thought that spending some of that money for aid to the poorest nations who have little or no hope in the future might, in the long run, be the best alternative to achieve peace in the world?

Intelligent questions need to be asked: Where are the terrorists that threaten the United States coming from? Where will they continue to come from? If underdeveloped nations are peopled by those with little or no hope for a better future, we can be sure there will be a series of terrorists from those nations for many years to come. The tragedy of September 11, 2001, was, in some respects, a wake-up call which we have been slow to analyze, except naively to declare that the criminals were guilty of envying our freedom. Our generous nation, built upon communitarian aid and compassionate sharing of our resources, responded this time with retaliatory violence in the name of protecting our national security. Would better results have been attained had we reached out with appropriate diplomacy and socioeconomic aid to those who have declared themselves our enemies? Critics of the political policies of the United States have claimed that our acts of vengeance and punishment of those we declare responsible for the attacks of September 11, 2001, have served only to further isolate ourselves from those hopeless, poverty-ridden nations where terrorists are recruited and trained. Were our nation to be more sensitive to the causes of terrorism and the worldwide injustices that continue to embitter the poor, we might be regarded by those same people as a living example of a moral nation instead of one that tends to shield itself from the world's suffering. But we are also living in a society that at present deems such questions and critical suggestions to be unpatriotic or even less supportive of the policies of retaliatory and preventive war now in vogue.

A SPIRITUALITY THAT RESPECTS ECOLOGY, THE ENVIRONMENT, AND RELATED HEALTH CARE ISSUES

As we were working on this segment of our book, Sudarsan Raghavan published an article in *The Philadelphia Inquirer* titled "From Man and Nature, Starvation." The article points out the effects of hunger and AIDS on millions of people in Southern Africa. The problem is not new. Hunger continues to torment the African continent in what seems like a conspiracy of disease, drought, political corruption, and wars that have crippled a once thriving agricultural production sufficient to feed the masses. Governmental cutbacks, the

AIDS pandemic, and hard-nosed debt-collection policies of First World banks, have also contributed to the misery that predicts to take the lives of over 16 million people per year in the near future.[16]

Raghavan laments that the Unites States news media, which could expose this worldwide crisis, has been obsessed, instead, with the war against Iraq and its consequences. The excitement of President George Bush's somber call to war evidently makes better copy than the suffering of millions of impoverished peoples in the developing world. The United States has cut back its development programs in aid to needy African nations to a third of what it used to spend during cold war days when competing with Russia for the natural resources of that continent.[17] The AIDS epidemic, from which some 28.5 million sub-Saharans suffer, has brought the African continent unimaginable anguish with work scarce, food even scarcer, and solutions as elusive as efforts to rebuild the village networks that in times past could provide for those otherwise bereft of the means for long-term survival.[18]

Ethicists have long argued that neglect of ecology and downplaying the importance of environmental concerns in favor of insuring economic prosperity for heavily industrialized, technologically advanced societies have contributed to present-day crises in health care on a global scale. In addressing this problem, many motives may intervene. A lasting solution involves more than the practical cleaning up of the environment out of concern for ecology and the improvement of peoples' health throughout the world. In addition to the practical benefits from more careful attention to ecology, we see the prime motivational force embedded in a spirituality that views nature and life itself as sacred. Faith in God dictates that we have special obligations toward our fellow human beings in terms of protecting the earth and the environments in which human life must thrive. Many of the rivers of the heavily populated nations are polluted. Potable water is scarce; several nations suffer from a chronic water shortage. The seas are now experiencing a sharp decline in the supply of fish. Several species have been found to be loaded with mercury and other toxins. With sources of food and water on the decrease, we have come face-to-face with the reality of our inability to produce indefinitely what humans in poverty need or what humans in their affluence demand.

THE WORLD'S DIMINISHING WATER SUPPLY:
A SOURCE OF ANXIETY AND POTENTIAL CONFLICT

Many areas of the world are, in fact, facing the dilemma of increasing demands for water in the midst of diminishing supply. Estimates reveal that there are 1 billion people in the world without sufficient supplies of potable water. Former U.S. Ambassador John McDonald, when assigned as U.S. Coordinator for the United Nations Oversight of Drinking Water and Sanitation, wrote the following:

> Nothing I had ever seen in my life prepared me for the day I landed in Africa. . . . people trekked miles in the hot sun just to get clean water for the day. But even more tragic were the children I saw suffering from the lack of clean water. Many seemed to be just hours from death, and others had lost their vision to trachoma, an easily preventable disease caused by contaminated water.[19]

Researchers claim that the lack of safe drinking water is the main cause of disease in the world, and about 40,000 people die from contaminated water every day across the globe. Over fifty nations suffer from water shortages, yet according to authorities involved in "Global Water," there is often ample water only 100 feet below the surface of many of these same countries. Organizations such as Global Water drill new wells and purify and store new and existing sources of water for domestic and agricultural use. But rural people can not dig by hand 100 feet below the ground to get to this water. This is where part of the problem and a possible solution lie.

The United Nations estimates that by the year 2015, 40 percent of the world's population will find it impossible, or at least very difficult, to obtain enough water for daily living purposes. This leads to the potential for conflict and violence over water rights and access. One example is the Euphrates River Valley where Turkey has been involved in damming the river upstream leaving a major problem down stream for Syria and Iraq.[20] Lebanon also is damming its water supply and thus cutting down the water going to Israel. Yet, in 1990, Israel desired to dam rivers in Ethiopia compelling Egypt to respond that this would be understood as an act of war.

Within our own country, south Texas farmers have evidently been able to access water from the Rio Grande by way of an agreement shared with Mexico. This has become a thorny issue because of a widespread drought in the Southwest. Water rationing in the Northeast U.S. has been a problem because of a lack of sufficient rain. It has been predicted that the Jordan River will dry up by 2015, and Lake Haroun in Iran, which is said to be the seventh largest freshwater lake, is now bone dry. Water is and will be an increasing global problem especially as the world's population continues to increase. This may become a major factor in triggering additional global violence. Critics say that some of the money spent in *future* space exploration might better be spent on *today's* water needs here and around the globe.

THE DANGER OF TOXINS IN DRINKING WATER

We take in toxins daily in the air we breathe, the water we drink, and the food we eat. The Physicians for Social Responsibility, an organization of over 20,000 physicians, health professionals, medical students, and citizens who have concerns about the destructive effects of nuclear weapons, worldwide violence, and issues related to environmental health for over forty years, are alarmed at this added danger to the health of the world. Gun violence, toxins in the air, water, and food are some of the issues that are on the agenda of this organization in its agitation for a safer world and for extending health care as a worldwide ministry. Even deeply set well water systems are affected. Some of the commonly found chemical toxins are pesticides, dioxins, furans, and PCBs (polychlorinated biphenyls). In addition, heavy metals such as lead and mercury linger on in their toxicity with no possibility for their biodegradation. Certain chemicals such as DDT and dioxin have even been found in human breast milk. They accumulate in fatty tissue and, when the fat reserves are depleted, the chemicals can pass through the placental barrier and harm the fetus.

The dangers from ordinary drinking water are connected to the costs of cleaning up the waterways of the world. But the people who continue to suffer from the toxins in their drinking water are, again, mainly the poor who lack either the financial means to detoxify their water or to engage in legal combat with the polluters. Yet, despite this bleak picture, a number of states have been able to engage in detoxifying strategies to purify their waters and to bring back an edible fishing population.

In that connection, a recent United Nations Human Development Report states that the richest one-fifth of the world amasses 82.7 percent of the world's income while the rest of the world can acquire only 17.3 percent of that income. "The scandal," according to Jesuit missionary Alberto Múnera, "is that the comfortable of the world live placidly (more or less) with the ticking time bomb of greedy consumption and ecological decay."[21] The ecological crisis that Múnera alludes to is as complex as a mosaic of interconnected pieces. James Nash, Executive Director of the Churches' Center for Theology and Public Policy in Washington, DC, lists these as the "pollution complex," comprising toxic pollution, global warming, and ozone depletion, all coupled with overpopulation, exhaustion of resources, maldistribution of resources, and the diminution and extinction of species. He adds "genetic engineering" to this list because of his ethical fear that this could lead to a misuse of technology and human power to shape nature without regard for the consequences. His analysis of pollution reads like a rogue's gallery of threats to human life against which morality should struggle: oil spills, ground-level ozone smog, hazardous biodischarges, acid rain, overexposure to radiation, pesticides, synthetic chemicals, noxious emissions, and metallic and other wastes. The list goes on to include dumped toxic chemicals in landfills as well as open dumps for garbage and solid wastes. The loss of health and life traceable to this pollution exposes the harm that neglect for ecology can do to the unsuspecting and susceptible.[22]

Nash's conclusion is worth noting in terms of how one's faith (or lack of it), one's moral sensitivity (or lack of it), can impinge on both health care issues and one's personal spirituality. "Poisoning our neighbors," he writes, "and wasting common commodities are not matters of privacy or free marketeering, or national sovereignty; they are serious moral offenses against others that demand public regulations and prohibitions."[23] Nash urges ethicists and those who set public policy for churches to denounce the polluters and to urge methods of sustaining an economy and an ecology that can promote both health and enhance the quality of human life on this earth. Most consumers, he observes, want the amenities and comforts of their modern home or life style without the poisonous by-products that in the longer run could threaten their life or long-term survival. The challenge to our spirituality, he argues, is to sustain the benefits from modern technology while doing away with its destructive side effects. He sees nature and grace not only as compatible but also as essentially complementary.[24] Nature need not always be bent to create the toxicity that emanates from high tech tactics of exploitation. In the same way, much as health care and prayer are compatible and to be encouraged, so too can ecological concerns and moral sensitivity be fused into one concern. Nature can be harnessed in a positive way to promote a healthier environment and an uplifting spirituality that will promote both good health and a healthy spirituality able to hail and preserve God's creation as good!

New critics of American-sponsored global economic dominance have emerged to question what has been presented as the inexorable economic laws of nations promoting the self-interests of its most powerful constituents. Theologian Rosemary Radford Ruether has attempted to focus her critical attention on the hard-nosed economic brokers of this world who support the global pursuit of self-interest by the rich and powerful that, in her opinion, has spawned massive unemployment, hunger, poverty, and destruction of the very earth on which we all depend. Opponents of the economic world order dictated by the affluent Western nations, she writes,

> are forming loose coalitions across social contexts. They are united in seeing the global system of corporate power, backed by the Bretton Woods institutions (the World Bank, International Monetary Fund, and the World Trade Organization) and American military supremacy, as shaping a new stage of world empire that is impoverishing the majority of humans and the earth while enriching a small elite of super rich.[25]

Ruether concludes that Christian theologians and their churches need to articulate an alternate vision that offers greater hope to the masses through structures and institutions that, unlike the Bretton Woods institutions, would feature an alternative vision to the present obscene system so inimical to the majority of the world's population, while favoring the mega affluent and politically well connected.

WAR AND THE WANTON DESTRUCTION
OF LIFE AND MORALITY

As we were writing this chapter, our nation's administration had completed what it prematurely called the "military phase" of its war with Iraq, a nation of 23 million people, 50 percent of whom are fifteen years old or younger, with the majority of its population living in poverty. Critics are divided on whether the reasons articulated for this "preventive war" have been compelling enough to have plunged the nation into a war that to many seemed not only unnecessary and illegal but also denounced by nearly every major religious body in the world.

The very horror of war should have been seen as not only a matter of concern for physicians and the health care ministry, but also as an important moral issue for theologians, ethicists, and religious people everywhere. Part of the problem is the way the Pentagon obscures the horrors of modern warfare. In his investigative analysis of how the opinions of the American public were influenced by the media and the administration, *Second Front: Censorship and Propaganda in the Persian Gulf War,* John B. MacArthur exposes the fraud behind the doublespeak terms "collateral damage," "precision bombing," and "surgical strike." These euphemisms hide the more hideous fact that bodies are torn to pieces, innocent civilians, women, old men, young children, and babies, are being killed.[26] MacArthur gives the media, "embedded" as they were with military units, a resounding "F" grade for its failure to properly investigate and criticize the language of deception perfected to mobilize public opinion in favor of the war. To hear the spokespersons of the Pentagon tell it, nobody, except demonized enemy military personnel, is really killed at the point where the bombs land.[27] George J. Bryjak of the University of San Diego challenges both politicians and the media not to call war anything other than "mass horror." His point is that "war movies, along with the politicians who send soldiers into battle, cannot or will not convey this horror, perhaps because so few of them have firsthand combat experience."[28]

Bryjak cites the military historian, Victor Davis Hanson, who had declared that for his fellow historians "to speak of war without vividly portraying the horrors of this enterprise 'is a near criminal offense.'" He challenges the media to show the suffering and to pester

Pentagon officials to report the truth about the lives of the innocent civilians destroyed in wartime. In cleverly withholding such information from the American public, the Pentagon seemed determined not to repeat their "mistake" in the Vietnam War. At that time the people could see firsthand television coverage of the bloodied casualties and body bags. This helped turn the public against the war. Even General Colin Powell proclaimed his lack of interest in Iraqi deaths—so much for compassion or for Jesus' mandate to love our enemies. Commenting on General Powell's attitude, Bryjak writes: "Little wonder, as the bodies of an estimated 300 to 500 women and children charred and mutilated beyond recognition after their bomb shelter was destroyed doesn't make for pleasant viewing on the nightly news."[29]

It is difficult for us to speak of the health care ministry without paying attention to the many thousands of people whose lives and health are threatened by modern warfare or by acts of violence both within nations culturally or ethnically divided, or by militaristic policies of superpowers seeking world dominance. Our purpose in this book is not to confine ourselves to the parochial interests of biomedical problems only within the United States. Both of us are strong believers in the Biblical teaching that we have been created in God's image and likeness and, thereby, we are committed to life and health issues beyond the borders of the United States. Both Doctors Without Borders and Physicians for Social Responsibility (PSR) have voiced their concerns that we include in our compassion the millions of people threatened by violence and oppression. Their lives are also valued in the eyes of the God whom we acknowledge as our divine caregiver. Many people in our nation find it difficult to remain silent when diplomatic dialogue has been abandoned in favor of the quick, easy solution of military intervention and the massive destructive bombing of targets that include civilians in a policy of total war.

What is particularly vexing to physicians and health care providers is the allied fact that the Department of Defense is allotted over a billion dollars a day to finance the most powerful military in the history of the world. The actual annual budget of nearly half a trillion dollars is six times that spent by Russia, the next largest spender in matters of national defense, and more than the next twenty-three nations combined. Pundits have declared that we are in a one nation arms race. On top of this outlandish outlay of funds for the military, there is a concomitant cut in the funds allocated for the alleviation of the sufferings of and care for the neediest of the citizens of this country. Theologian and former congressman Robert Drinan points out the senselessness of this national policy in an article denouncing the administration's unilateralism. He disputes the administration's assumption that the massive military power of the United States will keep American citizens safe. Drinan laments the United States' flaunting of the United Nations biological weapons convention, and its refusal to sign the treaty barring antipersonnel land mines, though every country in the western hemisphere except Cuba has signed it. He criticizes our withdrawal from the Kyoto Global Warming Treaty, as well as the refusal to ratify the International Criminal Court. Finally, he has serious doubts about the new doctrine of preemptive military action. These policy decisions have prompted several nations to accuse the United States of posturing itself, like a rogue nation, as above the rule of international law.

Drinan quotes former President Carter who has made the disparity between rich nations like the United States and the poorest people living in the underdeveloped nations a cause for concern by health care providers: "The results of this disparity are root causes of most of the world's unresolved problems, including starvation, illiteracy, environmental degradation, violent conflict and unnecessary illnesses, that range from Guinea worm to HIV/AIDS."[30]

VIOLENCE AS PROBLEM SOLVING: A MAJOR THREAT TO HEALTH

Mercy and justice, not advanced weaponry and massive killing of enemies, are the means incessantly mandated by the biblical word of God if people are ever to bring about a lasting peace in their world. The gift of forgiveness, and self-sacrificing love in the exercise of compassion has been constantly exemplified throughout Jesus' own ministry. The prophets are insistent that justice, including distributive justice for the poor, is required to eliminate oppression in its many forms, and thereby permit God's plan of peace to be fulfilled. In these crucial aspects of the biblical word and God's gift of faith are assumptions that people have been made aware that we are all children of God and must respect and be sensitive to each other's needs as well as the needs of our planet earth. Unfortunately power, greed, and self-aggrandizement can also be found among both individuals and nations. And these in turn are parent to the mistrust, misunderstanding, and chaotic violence that bring grief to the most vulnerable of the world's citizens. Social justice, if embraced as national policy, has the power to offset the pervasive force of criminality and oppression; it is only through justice that God's plan for God's people to live in peace with justice can become reality.

It goes without saying that most people would prefer negotiation and the nonviolent achievement of justice over against the brute force of military coercion. In this respect, most health care providers urge the passage of laws favoring peaceful solutions to political problems. But the dilemma remains as to just how effective would such laws be in a society constantly kept by its leaders in a state of fear and insecurity. The message proclaimed on a near daily basis by the administration and media is the overriding need to promote the ideology of national security, military force, and preventive war as the only path toward freedom from terrorism. The full impact of these policies on the poor of the United States has yet to be determined. What is certain, however, is that military expenditures drain away monies needed for social programs that benefit the needy.

The recently announced tax breaks to the wealthiest Americans in the face of budgetary deficits and a huge war debt have already consumed the budgetary surplus of not too long ago and threaten to destabilize programs for the poor and the chronically ill well into this century. As of this writing, many states and cities are financially unable to provide the services needed for adequate health care and other social services.

In this chapter we have enlarged the areas of our concerns to include an increased sensitivity to global injustice and poverty. Isolating the healing profession into the more narrow area of one's own town or country is impossible. The problems of this nation are connected on a global scale with the physical and mental torments suffered by people who are victims of war, hunger, personal degradation, and oppression. We have attempted to show that the United States, as the most powerful and affluent nation in the world, bears the larger responsibility to live up to its promise to promote the freedom and well-being of all peoples. The healing ministry should include working for justice and peace in areas scarred by pockets of suffering and despair.

To borrow from a letter of Dietrich Bonhoeffer written before his execution at Flossenbürg in April 1945, we must be people of prayer and action. The two go together. If health care providers pray with and for our patients, we must also be willing to engage in actions to promote justice and peace on both a national and international scale. The farewell words of Jesus Christ still hold: "Peace I leave with you; my peace I give to you. I do not give to you as the world gives" (John 14:27). Jesus offers the peace that derives from love, compassion, and forgiveness, even of enemies. The world offers only the false peace that comes through attacking, defeating and humiliating an enemy. The peace of God, not the peace that comes from war and killing of one's enemies, is religiously and socially responsible according to the dictates of a faith true to the respect for life at the heart of the religious traditions present in most of the nations of this world.

DISCUSSION QUESTIONS

1. Is the United States a sick society? Explain.
2. How do political policies impact on health care issues both positively and negatively?
3. Does the fact that the United States lacks universal health care and that over 45 million citizens have no medical insurance bode well for the American boast that the United States has the best medical system in the world? Explain.
4. Are political leaders unable to understand what the poor have to face in matters of destitution, hunger, and disease? Explain.
5. Comment on whether or how Bonhoeffer's statement can apply to health care providers.
6. Why is it so difficult for the affluent of societies to appreciate the problems in health care that the poor of the world face daily? How do we measure this against the moral teachings of Jesus Christ? Can we draw any moral conclusions from the disparity between bestowing tax breaks on the wealthiest of Americans and cutting programs for the poor and chronically ill?
7. What lessons for health and pastoral care of the needy can we draw from Jean Vanier's ministry in L'Arche? From the volunteer organizations Physicians for Social Responsibility and Doctors Without Borders?

8. Is there a connection between the failure of the nations to provide for their poor and the increase in acts of terrorism? Explain.

9. Comment on the following: It may be that the term *globalization* should not always be construed as a "vicious monster" chewing up the planet to the disadvantage of the depressed world and aggrandizement of those in the industrialized world. Author Peter Paris believes communities need such strong individuals as Desmond Tutu, Nelson Mandela, and Martin Luther King Jr. to uphold the universal moral and spiritual values of justice and peace without which the dreaded monster could very well gobble up the planet.[31]

10. Can we form an opinion on the impact of United States military actions on health and pastoral care?

Chapter 9

Healing Services:
Miracles, Cures, and Hope

God hears our prayers for healing and, at such times, some form of healing always occurs. We have tried to distinguish between healings and cures, particularly in the case of terminal illness. Even in cases of the terminally ill, a healing is always possible, but dramatic cures of physical maladies are rare occurrences attesting to the free and unpredictable intervention of God into our everyday lives. Often, too, what occurs at healing services can, indeed, seem miraculous. In this chapter we will report on many such services and their impact on those who yearn in hope for the medical cures that have eluded them. Some of these come to a service hoping only to experience healing of their spiritual and emotional ills rather than a cure of their physical maladies.

The earliest church record of an "official" healing service appears in the Epistle of James the Apostle. James was urging on the churches a practice that undoubtedly originated with the Apostles who healed in the manner of Jesus, whose teachings they followed. We read James' advice in the matter of dealing with illness. Sick people, he says, should pray. But he adds:

> Are any among you sick? They should call for the elders of the church and have them pray over them, anointing them with oil in the name of the Lord. The prayer of faith will save the sick, and the Lord will raise them up; and anyone who has committed sins will be forgiven. Therefore confess your sins to one another, and pray for one another, so that you may be healed. The prayer of the righteous is powerful and effective. (James 5:14-16)

James's advice is very close to Jesus' commissioning his disciples "to cure every kind of disease and every sickness" (Matthew 10:1).

Is There a God in Health Care?
© 2006 by The Haworth Press, Inc. All rights reserved.
doi:10.1300/5554_09

One may wonder whatever happened over the long span of church history to the kind of healing that James seemed to think was commonplace in his day. One phenomenon that seemed to replace the services that directly petitioned the Lord to rescue the sick from their illness was the cult of the saints. The revered holy person could effect the cure and that in itself would prove that the saint was truly in heaven, exercising great power of curative persuasion with the Lord. Those were the miracles that even today constitute in the Catholic Church the "proof" of sanctity prior to the actual canonization ceremony in the Basilica of Saints Peter and Paul in Rome.

Yet healing services abound today and those gifted with healing powers are not endeavoring to attain the high honor of canonization. Far from it! Sometimes the healings are integrated into the regular life of a church community on the assumption that every one of us at one time or another has need of inner peace and well-being. And this, in turn, may depend on the acknowledgement of our sins coupled with the experience of forgiveness. At other times, such services are offered for people who suffer from illnesses that may vary from a chronic sickness, to nagging mental depression, or even to those who may have been diagnosed as terminally ill. Some have described their experiences in these services as a genuine encounter with the annealing power of God or coming in touch with the healing power of Jesus Christ as embodied in the actions and prayers of a saintly person through whom God has chosen to work a "miracle." One such healing priest, the Reverend Ralph DiOrio, is insistent that he does not heal and that neither God nor he are "faith healers." From the perspective of a believing physician, the medical ministry calls for doctors to counter the illness with all the "weapons" at their disposal, then step back, and let God do the healing.

This nuance is important for Father DiOrio. He counsels those who come to him seeking a "cure" to continue to follow their medical treatments. He explained what happens within him in those instances of healing that occur during the services that are structured into his ministry to the sick.

> Jesus, the Divine Physician, out of his compassion and love for us, knows our needs, hears our calls, and heals. I am simply a conduit through which he sends his healing love. Why or how God chose me, I do not know, but I sincerely thank him and accept his will for me. I also cannot tell you why or how God

selects whom or what illness he will and will not heal, except that he does not base the decision on the amount of the person's faith.[1]

Father DiOrio's amazing record of healings both physical and spiritual led the Diocese of Worcester to appoint him the Director of its Healing Ministry. The book, which contains convincing attestations of the healings attributed to the interventions of this remarkable priest, is filled with stories, highlighting the medical background of each particular case, and the dramatic breakthrough to healings through some action or word of his.

Two of the healings attributed to Father DiOrio's intercession are noteworthy. The case of Barbara MacRae defied all medical expectations. Barbara had been diagnosed as suffering from an inflammatory cancer of the breast that had already spread to the lymph nodes and spine. Chemotherapy was prescribed. She was also told that there was little hope, given the aggressive nature of this kind of cancer. But they had an experimental treatment that involved forty-nine other people with the same kind of cancer. These patients would be bombarded with cancer-killing drugs. The treatment seemed worse than the cancer itself. Though totally exhausted, she was able to go to Father DiOrio's service at St. John's Church in Worcester. After his announcement that he was going to minister to the sick as the Holy Spirit moved him to do so, he called out to those in attendance: "There is a woman here who is being healed of breast cancer and she is dressed in black and white. Would she please stand up."[2] Because her colors were blue and white, she hesitated to stand up.

Finally, Father DiOrio kept calling until he asked that every woman suffering from breast cancer stand up. At that point some fifty women stood up. But he pointed at Barbara and said out loud, "It's you, honey! Come around here."[3] She was asked if she believed in the power of the Holy Spirit. On her answer that she did so believe, he asked her to close her eyes and thank Jesus. A feeling of deep contentment came over her and she seemed to be impelled toward a beautiful light. She was told to go back from that light. She woke up lying on the floor. Rising from the floor with great ease, she felt that the cancer was gone. All the pain had likewise disappeared.[4] Subsequent X-rays and a bone scan revealed no signs of the cancer. Still, the doctors insisted that she go through the full treatment. Two years after the therapy was terminated she was told that she was the only survivor of the entire test group. All the others had died. Barbara continues to call this "the gift of new life."[5] Some speculate that the inner peace from the healing service may have triggered amazing strength to her immune system.

Even more amazing is the story of the medical doctor, Alberto Barrera, who had been a surgeon and a medical practitioner for forty-five years and who, though he believed in God's guidance during his surgery, was skeptical about the wonders attributed to Father DiOrio. He has described his troubles as beginning in 1977 with chest pain caused by angina that grew with increasing intensity for the next several years. On each admission to the CCU of the hospital, his own colleagues dismissed his troubles as nothing more than anxiety neurosis. He began to treat himself with nitroglycerin, even in the face of the medical dictum that "the doctor who treats himself has a fool for a patient and an idiot for a doctor." On his seventh admission in 1984, he demanded a thallium scan of his heart. This time the test showed a serious blockage of four coronary arteries. A subsequent angiogram confirmed that this to be the case, necessitating coronary bypass. This intervention gave him only eighteen months of pain-free existence. Once again he began to deteriorate, having failed a stress test, and after another angioplasty, he learned that one of the bypasses was completely blocked. His heart developed a serious rhythm disturbance during the procedure, requiring several defibrillator shocks before his heart began to beat more regularly again. Further surgery was deemed too risky.

After his discharge, he frequently needed to use an oxygen mask, increased nitroglycerin, and either morphine or Demerol to relieve the pain. With his oxygen tanks in tow, he consulted the head cardiologist at Yale and was told that, beyond painkillers, there was nothing else that could be done for him. He returned home resigned to his death and set about putting his affairs in order. But after collapsing and being taken again to the hospital, his wife told him she was taking him to see Father DiOrio. Still suspicious and skeptical, he tried to find out about this priest. A Massachusetts state trooper, a self-proclaimed atheist, told him that he did not "know how much the church paid these guys to pretend they were healed." So, not believing in "that DiOrio fellow" he decided to go with his wife just to please her. He set out with his wife, son, and five tanks of oxygen in 1986. His diffidence continued on entering the auditorium. He admitted thinking, *So here is a man walking around waving his arms. Oh no, not another one of those revival meetings where people roll on the ground!* As he put it, "I arrived at the service with one percent belief and 99 percent disbelief." Despite his doubts, he prayed "Lord, if I am wrong to disbelieve, forgive me and help me to believe."[6]

When Father DiOrio blessed him on the forehead, Dr. Barrera felt a calm come over him, but was surprised when Father DiOrio stopped and rushed back to him and with his face very close to the doctor told him, "You have work yet to do." The statement sounded preposterous, given his age and infirmity. But soon he was able to take off his oxygen mask, walk up the incline to a level spot, take seven steps, and still be able to breathe. He then surprised everybody including himself by walking to his car and announcing that he was going to drive. He no longer felt the need for oxygen, pain medication, or heart medicine. Only one setback loomed on his horizon: he had to undergo withdrawal from his addiction to the pain medication. But the good news intensified when an additional thallium scan revealed that there were no longer any dark areas in his heart. Not long after that scan he was able to go swimming and dancing. His final remark is worth noting, given his earlier skepticism: "I thank God and Father DiOrio for my life, and I will continue to use it to serve God."[7]

The conversion from skeptic to believer in the matter of seemingly miraculous cures and healings is not unique. In fact, the celebrated healer Emily Gardiner Neal described herself as a religious skeptic with a closed mind locked against the possibility of Christian healing. Her journey to belief in the powers of spiritual healing is documented in her book *A Reporter Finds God Through Spiritual Healing.*[8] Her journey began on a cold evening in February, when she was asked by a new neighbor to drive him to an important meeting at 8:00 that night. She agreed but reluctantly, since she scarcely knew this man and she was busy writing at the time and the roads were icy and dangerous. He explained to her that his little daughter was in the hospital with meningitis and he hoped to attend the healing service to pray for her so she would be helped. For Emily, this was nonsense talk, compounded by the fact that he was going to the Episcopal Church which she imagined was too "ultradignified" to be doing "healing services." The weather worsened, but they made it to the church, and Emily, not wanting to while away the time in her car, went inside. There she saw a woman with an enormous goiter. The service began with a hymn and prayer followed by a short talk on spiritual healing by the priest who pointed out that Christ had commissioned his church to preach the kingdom and also to heal, the two commands being inseparable. She felt terribly out of place. This was not the Jesus she had revered as a great teacher of ethical behavior and moral leadership. She closed her eyes, but then the priest was summoning those who sought healing to present themselves at the altar for healing and communion. She watched them file by, noticing a young lad whose hands were covered with warts.

Emily's misgivings began to diminish as the atmosphere seemed to be filled with a very "palpable faith" and she started to pray that God not let all those trusting people down. "Please don't let them down, but honor their faith."[9] Only later would she note the incongruity of her, an unbeliever, praying to a God in whose existence she had no faith. She could feel the heat emanating from the woman sitting beside her. Her neighbor friend also returned with tears in his eyes and a look of great joy. Emily could not help thinking about what might happen if his daughter had died during the service.

At the end of the service she could see that the goiter on the woman she had noticed earlier had completely disappeared and so too the warts on the young boy's hands. Was it a dream or was she losing her mind? She drove her neighbor to the hospital and went about her writing assignment; however, she could not drive from her mind the "cures" she had witnessed. Were they merely psychosomatic cures? Also, she was filled with suspense about her neighbor's daughter so she phoned him. He thanked her for taking him to the church service, and he added that his daughter was well. "They can't understand at the hospital what happened—that is, nobody but our doctor can. Funny thing, but he doesn't seem surprised."[10] Later, Emily had lunch with her doctor. He was also the new neighbor's doctor. The doctor then described what had happened: "Remarkable recovery that child made. We'd done all we could do for her medically. Scientifically speaking, she didn't have a chance—but now she's fully recovered. You could almost say it was a miracle." The doctor added that he had seen a woman who had been scheduled to have a goiter operation today but, after the healing service, the goiter had spontaneously disappeared. It was the same woman that Emily had noticed in the beginning of the church service. This was the beginning of Emily's attending many more healing services in various churches in order to reinforce her newly discovered convictions about the ministry of healing. Eventually, she would be called to her own healing ministry and become a leading spokeswoman for the healing movement itself.[11]

THEOLOGIAN GEFF'S PERSONAL EXPERIENCE IN A HEALING SERVICE

My own bout with the kind of skepticism that Emily Gardiner Neal experienced came during a healing service conducted by Father DiOrio. The experience of my daughter's healing was not too dissimilar to that described by Doctor Barrera. We had heard of those "miracles" attributed to Father DiOrio at the time when the hospital had told us that our daughter was terminally ill. Even after her many surgeries, chemotherapy, and radiation, the tumor was again mushrooming and was posing a serious threat to her life. But we refused to put her back on chemotherapy because of the previous trauma of her near death, intense pain, and the fact that the side effects of the proposed protocol included possible deafness and blindness. Our decision was to focus on two of Susan's greatest joys—music and meeting people. We told the doctor that we would fill her heart with love and care in the remaining time she had to live, but we could not in conscience submit her to another bout with the destructive chemicals that might counteract the effects of the tumor but make her life miserable. The hospital contacted the Make-A-Wish Foundation, and so what looked like Susan's last year of life began with an unforgettable trip for the whole family to DisneyWorld where we enjoyed a week of forget-all-your-troubles fun.

Looking back on those days and keeping up with the news of those terminally ill children then being granted their wish with Susan to visit DisneyWorld, it is sad to report that nearly all of them are dead or, in the words of the foundation, have joined the "stars of heaven."

Attending healing services to support a friend or some blood relation not in the immediate family is one thing. At that time, if there is not a familial closeness or an intimacy in the friendship, say, of a friend or neighbor, prayer and faith may come more easily. But to pray and hope that a beloved family member, especially one's own child, be completely "cured" through a "miracle" occurring at a healing service where so many such "miracles" have taken place for others can be much more difficult.

With little hope for Susan's cure, we thought we had nothing to lose if we took her to be touched by Father DiOrio. We had heard of Father DiOrio, not just from his book, but also through word-of-mouth. Previously, I had tried to contact another healing priest closer to home, Father Joseph Orsini, who had been recommended by a priest of the Diocese of Camden whom I met at an ordination ceremony. Susan was with us and, at some twenty-six pounds, looked sick and skeletal. The priest urged me to contact Father Orsini. I was able to contact his secretary who described to me how Father Orsini had been instrumental in his being personally healed of a life-threatening cancer. He also informed me of the scheduled healings and the community services during which such prayers for healings would take place. None of these services corresponded with times when either I was free or Susan was not at the hospital. Finally, I succeeded in making a telephone connection with Father Orsini. I told him of my inability to connect with his prayer community and then asked if I could bring Susan to him at his rectory. His reply was interesting. "Geff," he said, "you can bring her to me anytime but I must tell you that no 'cure' will take place. If I had the power you think I have, I'd be in the hospitals every day working those 'wonders.' The healings take place only during the prayer services of our community. It seems the only time when the healing power of God does what you are hoping and praying for."[12] I resolved to take Susan to one of those services.

The prospect of taking her to Father DiOrio's service became a reality when the parents of a student of mine, who had died suddenly from an unsuspected aneurysm at age nineteen, offered to drive us to Massachusetts. They wanted to bring their overwhelming grief to Father DiOrio in hopes of some assurance about their son and some positive healing of their grief. We then drove to Sturbridge, Massachusetts, where Father DiOrio's ministry had rented the ballroom of a local hotel to accommodate over a thousand people from that section of the state. These people had crowded into the makeshift space already set up with a portable altar readied for the Mass, which would take place after lunch. I was bringing to this service my innate theologian's skepticism, but not a little hope that something would happen to help Susan. Doctors in their scientific training and theologians in their rigid theological formation tend to be skeptical of claims that a "miracle" had taken place. The mainstream churches are themselves diffident about visions, sightings of the Blessed Virgin in some park or shrine, tears from a statue, or voices heard by someone certifiably neurotic. None of these bizarre claims were present in any of the healing services I have ever attended, but that skepticism was certainly present during my drive to Sturbridge.

Because Susan was in a wheelchair at the time—it was just after another of her shunt revision surgeries—she was ushered up front with the babies, children, and others in wheelchairs. I was not expecting the free-and-easy way in which Father DiOrio eventually entered the ballroom, greeting people, waving, and looking both relaxed and friendly. He said words of greeting to all those in attendance. He then went over to the babies and children and those who were wheelchair bound in the first rows and began prayers of healing. The prayers were individual and dreamlike. I watched Father DiOrio's face intently, looking for signs of satisfaction or of disappointment. Finally, Susan's turn came. He placed his hands on her head and prayed. But his face seemed dour with disappointment. He placed a small crucifix in her hands and gave me a look of futility before passing on to the next child. There it was, for me, the proof that nothing would happen. I was mistaken!

During the morning prayer services, Father DiOrio often paused and went into a kind of trance. He would then mention that someone in the audience was troubled with stomach problems or some other illness that he detected. The sick person's name or a description of the person was then spoken and he or she was asked to come forward. I looked around and on one of those summons I could see the man's wife pushing him up and out of the row of seats. Father DiOrio would then address the man (or woman) publicly and describe what he sensed was the trouble, be it a cancer, a crippling arthritis, or a host of other troubles. He would then ask the person to believe in the power of the Holy Spirit to heal and then pray over the person while laying on hands. At times, he would tell a person to remove his or her hearing aid. In another instance, a woman in a wheelchair was asked to stand up. She did. It was a truly intriguing ceremony for even a theological skeptic such as me. I saw healings taking place before my eyes. I saw faith and hope evinced as never before, but I still privately wondered why such power could not be channeled to help my daughter. This went on with Father DiOrio sometimes going into a trance, or breaking out in prayer, or offering reflections on God's mercy. At other times he urged the people not to abandon either their physicians or their medicines and not to think that healings were other than the work of God. It is God who heals, although not always in the manner we would like.

At the lunch break, a friend who had been in my wife's prayer group and who had moved to Massachusetts insisted that I meet with Father DiOrio since he was very interested in Dietrich Bonhoeffer and I had brought my first book on Bonhoeffer with me as a gift. Father had just come from a group of petitioners for whom he had laid on hands and offered prayers for healing. He reached his hand out to me and I to him, but his hand was as hot as a steaming iron and I wanted to scream. I recoiled my hand and he apologized for not having realized the intense heat that his laying on of hands generated. We had a little chat about Bonhoeffer and I presented my book to him.

The Mass began in the early afternoon, interrupted sporadically by a spontaneous healing moment. His homily was not brilliant by any means, but I do remember the compassion with which he spoke, and the loving way he lauded God's strange mercy. At the communion, while I was wheeling Susan to the front to receive the host, Father DiOrio seemed to go into another of his trances. He put the ciborium (sacred cup) on the altar and went directly to Susan and laid his hands on her and prayed intensely over her. Surprised, I could only watch his face. I saw a calm and a look of pleasure come over him. My heart beat faster and I received the communion with Susan and my wife, who was standing beside me.

Not long after that, the next brain scan revealed that the tumor had not grown. Every brain scan after that to this day has shown the tumor's growth completely arrested. The tumor, reduced in size, still sits on her brainstem, but Susan continues to experience relatively good health. A couple of years after she went into spontaneous remission, Susan was taken off seizure medicine on an experimental basis and, at this writing, she has not had any more seizures. The doctors have been both pleased and amazed at her progress. Can we call this a "miracle" or a healing? Most "cures" are really only reprieves for reasons known to God alone. Whatever happened on that day in Sturbridge, Massachusetts, I am no longer a skeptic when it comes to the healing services through which a chronic illness is reversed or terminal illness seemingly arrested, when broken hearts are suddenly mended, when sick children recover although no further medical intervention was possible.

HEALING SERVICES: WITH OR WITHOUT FAITH

Healing services have become appreciated more and more. So, too, are texts that describe the varying modes of the healing ministries available to people everywhere. Several documented "cures" range from the spectacular throwing away of crutches, to instantaneous disappearance of cancers, to recuperation from a crippling arthritis, to the more simple alleviation of unbearable pain, and many other recoveries from illness. Those who have visited the shrines of Saint Anne de Beaupré or the sainted Brother André of Montreal cannot fail to notice the huge piles of crutches, wheelchairs, eyeglasses, hearing aids, testimonials of miraculous cures through the intercession of these saints, the grandmother of Mary, or the humble layman noted for his piety. A visit to Lourdes or other religious shrines yields the same testimonials to the ever-present power of God to heal the sick and cure the so-called "incurable."

Wherever prayer services of healing exist, hopes for alleviation or even a "cure" will continue to be encouraged. Although healers such as Kathryn Kuhlman have testified that healings can take place without faith, Dominican priest Francis MacNutt, who has been very active in healing ministries both in the United States and Latin America, speculates that "perhaps such healings are meant by God to help people receive the faith they do not yet have."[13] Yet both are insistent that faith is important for healing, although MacNutt adds that "God will bless us far beyond our own merits. . . . We need to take ourselves less seriously—and God more seriously."[14] The danger is that when a "cure" does not take place, people may begin to blame themselves for their lack of faith or for having an unworthy disposition.

MacNutt cautions against those services that promise deliverance but, because of the pressures of determining whether one's faith was sufficient, generate their own fear and anxiety. He cites Kathryn Kuhlman who has herself asked why some people are cured of their infirmity while others are as sick afterward as before or even worse off, from a medical standpoint. Her reply is helpful in arriving at a sane balance to theological assumptions that pretend to know the mind of God and the inner psychic strength of a believer:

> I have decided that God doesn't have preferences in theology. We are the ones who try to put a fence around God, to bring him down to our level. But it doesn't work. God is too big for us to confine. . . . I'm still learning the mysterious ways in which God moves. I'll tell you one thing—I'm sure God has a sense of humor.[15]

Kuhlman recounts how she was theologically shaken when a person who claimed he had no faith at all was cured of his deafness at a service. At the time, Kathryn had believed that the process of healing could be so structured that healings would naturally occur. Ever since that experience, she would admit publicly that she did not know why some with admirable faith are not healed. "Healing is mysterious," she wrote. "The best that man can do is to bow down before the mystery that is God."[16]

DOCTOR BILL'S PERSONAL REFLECTIONS ON HEALING SERVICES

In a case very similar to the healings Geff has described, I remember a healing service that took place during an annual retreat for Third Order Franciscans held at Greymoor, the home of First Order Franciscans, located in Garrison, New York. In this instance, a middle-aged lady, also a Third Order Franciscan from Princeton, wished for healing of a painful and crippling hip disorder. Several of us present placed our hands on the affected area during the service. Following this service, she no longer required a cane, regained a normal gait, had lost the discomfort in the area, and enjoyed this state for several years. We all agreed that, at times, a group of believers can release a saturation of God's power and become instruments in bringing about God's immediate response for reasons known only to God alone.

Interest is growing in conducting healing services in the mainlline churches. These services are far from uniform and vary among different groups and churches. Healing services in our local church are held at the end of the 11:15 a.m. service on Sundays, and also Wednesdays at 5:30 p.m. "Special times" or occasions for healing services are also held, but these are not done on a regular basis.

These services may play a role in church renewal as more individuals seek respite and release from their physical and emotional hurts. They can also serve as a potential mechanism for interdenominational Christian healing and a step toward ecumenical church unity. The sufferings of humanity transcend the denominational divisions that have bedeviled Christianity over its history. The need for a compassionate ministry to the suffering among us offers an opportunity for all Christians, despite their dogmatic or liturgical differences, to establish a common bond in works of mercy. We must not lose sight of the fact that the church body represents the Body of Christ in the many forms that this body exhibits. This includes all peoples in its compassionate outreach, despite their dogmatic and liturgical differences.

Laying on of Hands

In many healing services among the "mainline" churches, where the context is a Eucharistic service, it is recommended that the anointing or laying on of hands with prayers for the troubled individual take place before the Eucharist. Healing prayers that seem appropriate can include reading from various biblical sources, such as James 5:14-16 or Psalm 23. A passage from the Gospel, perhaps John 6:47-51 ("I am the bread of life"), is also read. The Eucharist is presided over by the priest. A healing blessing usually concludes the church service. Following the blessing, lay ministers are commissioned to bring the sacraments to the hospital, home or hospice. Many patients are mentioned and prayed for during the intercessions that precede the Eucharistic prayers.

From our perspective, however, the prayers and laying on of hands very often occurs beyond the church walls and not necessarily as part of a healing service. I have done hands-on prayers in auditoriums, parking lots, house calls, and wherever the need for prayerful healing has been requested. In all cases and locations it helps to know the diagnosis before starting prayers for a return to physical or spiritual wholeness. The diagnosis and the stage of the illness determine the direction of the prayer. Also, the prayers themselves should be considered to be Spirit-led, that is, we should acknowledge our trust in

God knowing that we are only instruments in the healing power of the Holy Spirit dwelling in both the healer at prayer and the person in need of the help.

Power is found in a group of people in their laying hands on a person who is suffering. This is difficult to prove, but it makes sense to us. We have found this to be true in our own experiences. "Death to self," which can occur in group prayer, may open the door wider to the Spirit's healing powers. Group prayer creates an enormous amount of caring and dynamism flowing through all present, as they lay hands on someone in need. In 1981, while on a retreat in Florida, twelve people placed their hands on me and prayed. I could feel the healing power coming through them. I will always remember it.

A Healing Service in the ICU

I hope it is clear that healing services can occur within, as well as outside the actual church building, even within the ICU of our hospital. Helen, a seventy-three-year-old patient, had sustained a fractured hip from a fall a number of years prior. She elected to have hip surgery in a metropolitan hospital. The surgery went well except for her being placed on a ventilator postoperatively for a couple of days. Helen also required a transfusion of a couple of units of blood. When in my office, following her discharge, she had only one major complaint, and it was the possibility of being placed on an assisted breathing machine following the surgery. This had upset her emotionally. She made me promise never to allow this to happen in the future as she admitted to being claustrophobic. So, on her insistence, I wrote "No ventilator" in her chart.

A blood test report about three years after her hip surgery was found to be positive for HIV (human immunodeficiency virus), most likely from tainted blood in the transfusion following surgery. This was a time when AIDS had become a new medical entity in our country. The consensus at that time was not to treat Helen since she seemed free from any other symptoms. One Saturday evening, however, she was admitted to the ICU with a fever of 103 degrees, cyanotic lips, pneumonia involving both lungs, and marked shortness of breath. Despite being barely alert, she still reminded me of my promise to avoid a ventilator. She was deathly ill and really required a ventilator. Blood gases showed very low oxygen and high carbon dioxide levels in her circulation, which undoubtedly contributed to her confusion and agitation. By thrashing about, she was using up her already low oxygen level, vitally important for all of her body tissues and organs. Her condition rapidly deteriorated; blood tests revealed a continual decline of oxygen levels and rise in carbon dioxide levels.

Because of her refusal of a ventilator, our options were limited. An early attempt to place an oxygen pressure mask over her face was ineffective. Restraints made her struggle all the more and only aggravated the situation. Sedatives would only depress the respiratory center in the medulla. Meantime, cultures were taken and antibiotics were given. The curtains around her bed were drawn. Three of us worked as fast as possible: a pulmonary technician, a nurse with a dove on her name tag (a symbol of both the Holy Spirit and peace), and myself. I asked Helen if we could pray for her and she agreed. The nurse and technician, when asked, also wanted to participate. We then placed our hands on Helen's head and shoulders and prayed into her ear that God was present and would give her the needed peace to relax, stop struggling, and "let go." Soon after the prayer, and remaining at her side, we noted the struggling began to decrease! We continued to watch her closely over the next few hours. To our great joy, her color and blood oxygen levels started to improve. It seemed she might make it! The mental confusion lessened, and her agitation ceased. Five days later, she was well enough to be transferred from the ICU to a step-down unit. Not too many days later, Helen was discharged and sent home.

In prior years I would have said, "She was lucky." But now I say she was "fortunate." God had intervened. Having exhausted all medical possibilities, and with no other means of treatment available, prayer made the difference. She was able to "let go," to surrender, and God took over the healing. To this day I do not know if she had a specific religious commitment to any denomination, but we do know that God loves all of God's children. Our trio of health caregivers at her bedside will always remember the remarkable recovery from her devastating AIDS pneumonia and the power of prayer that played such a crucial role in her recovery.

In the early 1980s, I took part in another unique healing service that became a new experience for me. Sister Miriam Murphy, who by chance wound up being my spiritual director, suggested I go to the tenth annual Charismatic Conference at Notre Dame University. A devout nun of the Order of Notre Dame, she was both an ecumenist and a spiritual director with a gift for healing. She led me on, and I soon found myself among 10,000 people with their arms raised up and praising God in song—a strange happening that reminded me of similar actions by parishioners in the Assembly of God parish in Princeton led by my friend, the Reverend Jesse Owens. It was an important adjunct for the healing process to be a less uptight Christian in order to be more open to God's presence, and as I later found out to be more open to my patients as well. After all, I had been schooled always to use the science aspect of my medical training. The only arm-raising I had done had to do with exercise and physical therapy. No one ever mentioned the word "God," or anything pertaining to a patient's soul or spirit. What a surprise to find myself in the midst of Catholic priests, monsignors, other members of the hierarchy, and laypeople, all of whom I expected to be as uptight as I was—and they were not! The service had a bonding, unifying effect, a community of believers rejoicing as one voice. Although I knew no one, there was a feeling of oneness. I returned home and felt good that the scientific brick wall that had surrounded me for twenty years was crumbling and being replaced by a new and wonderful openness. An inner healing was well on its way. The location of this particular church service happened to be an outdoor stadium.

Another friend of mine, Father Gerald Ruane, has spent the great majority of his priesthood using his gift of healing and is still going strong. He began the Sacred Heart Institute of Healing in Northern New Jersey a few decades ago, and I was privileged to be a participant in some of his church healing sessions. On one occasion, twelve of us were in line in the back of a church near the New Jersey shore. Father Gerry worked his way down the line praying individually for each of us. Everyone he touched became "filled with the Spirit" and fell backward. There were men stationed behind each person being prayed for, who were able to catch those who might fall. I remember lying on my back, looking up at the ceiling, experiencing a deep sense of peace.

On a different occasion, at the conclusion of a seashore weekend retreat, and before leaving for our respective homes, Father Ruane led us to an empty schoolyard where we watched as two school buses arrived with mainly elderly folks who disembarked and formed four lines. We were to offer prayers for their healing. Their faith-filled trust in God's healing power was the driving force that brought them to this location. Many used canes or crutches. Some appeared to be suffering from a variety of handicaps. A couple of us stood at the head of each of the four lines of those seeking healing prayers. One by one they came, and for each one separately we prayed for a healing. Tears came to my eyes as I witnessed the strong faith of these suffering people. It was awesome for me to realize I was that afternoon being used as one of God's instruments for healing. For me, it was powerful stuff! Today, many years later, I know for sure God hears our prayers and always brings some noticeable healing—but not always a physical cure.

A Healing Service in Prison

My own experience of being healed led me to experience a new avocation, that of not only lecturing on the importance of prayer in the health care professions, but also making myself available for healing services to which friends invite me. This led me one day to an experience of healing I as a physician would never have dreamed of. This was the time the late Sister Retzie Piper, a Sacred Heart nun, asked me to join her for one of her discussion groups and healing services as part of her prison ministry. Sister Retzie would ask individuals to give talks to prisoners usually on what that person's vocation was like, in my case that of a physician. But this was unknown territory and a challenge to me that I will never forget. What could I say that might bring healing into the lives of these lonely inmates of a state prison?

Upon passing through the main entrance there then followed the horrible clanging noise as two sliding steel gates closed beyond us. We handed over our wallets. We were then led down a hall to a room with a desk and chairs arranged in a semicircle. I noticed a guard pacing back and forth in the hall after he had made sure there was no ruckus. We entered the room and saw twenty inmates sitting in the semicircle of chairs, waiting for us. The prisoners were quite young, their ages ranging from twenty to thirty-five years. They were talking with each other; a little shoving was going on and some tough talk, but no serious problems of behavior. After saying a few words, Sister introduced me. I asked the Lord to speak through me as I related my own journey, touching upon my unexpected loss, my loneliness, my eventual healing which had led me to a new appreciation of the power of shared prayer.

My talk went on for about thirty minutes, during which time I was able to give a number of examples of healing in working with my patients. At the end I reminded them that we were special people regardless of our backgrounds and that God loves us despite our failings. I mentioned we all have different gifts; they had gifts that I did not have and I had some they did not have. Sister interjected her comments as well. At the end of our allotted time I was shocked to see how silent and interested they had become. Was the Holy Spirit able to touch some of them with God's healing power merely through our sharing of experiences? It seemed appropriate to ask them to stand, clasp hands, and pray for the spiritual healing we all need. After praying for them, Sister found a blank sheet of paper in the desk drawer and said we would pray for the healing of each one present by his first name in the next few weeks, if they so wished. They were invited to come forward and sign their first names on the sheet of paper. I remember all but two or three came forward. They were prayed for at home in subsequent healing services.

We then retraced our steps, retrieved our wallets, heard once again the ominous clang of the two steel sliding doors, and went to the car. What did we reflect upon as we drove away? The inmates had demonstrated both an interest in prayer and a hunger for the healing prayers that would be offered on their behalf. They were able to become vulnerable by holding one another's hands in prayer as well as coming forward to write their first names to request follow-up healing prayers. They appeared to be genuine people, who had made mistakes in life. The Holy Spirit's healing presence was undoubtedly present in that room. The dreadful clanging made by the steel doors closing behind us will continue to haunt me for a long time.

I witnessed another kind of suffering and a new pathway for spiritual healing. Sister Retzie's prison ministry was her gift from the Lord to those inmates. They were isolated from society, out of view, and so easily forgotten by us all, yet, as the Gospels never cease to remind us, one with us in the Lord and among the least of Jesus' brothers. Jesus said: "I was in prison and you came to visit me" (Matthew 25:36). This was a powerful experience for me; one that I will long remember. It served once again to illustrate my growing conviction that the Lord does indeed speak through us in the various healing ministries to which we have been called. The power of God's providential healing of his children must extend into even the darkest recesses of human existence where people are often among society's outcasts and throwaways and, yes, even those serving time or languishing on death row in depressing prisons both here and abroad.

In their ministry of healing, many of the churches in the early years of the United States were among the first to build hospitals. The religious who founded these institutions desired both medical care as well as the provision for the spiritual needs of the patients. This reinforced the importance of healing the whole person. Even today, the presence of chaplains, available for in-house services and hands-on prayer, carry on the church's tradition going back to Jesus' ministry of healing and teaching. Following hospital discharge, the patient's spiritual and medical needs continued to be addressed, again under the caring mission of both the church and the attending physician.

As we are engaged on our respective journeys back to God, our prayer life often demands a balance between two forces. The first emanates from our need to serve God. The second is, as the occasion presents itself, to offer intercessory prayers for those in need both within church services and beyond the perimeters of any one church; people are hurting as much today as in the past. Patients are more likely to ask for prayers, or at least an extra moment for the caregiver's attentive ear. They want to know that God is present and that God will heal them in mind, body, and spirit as was true throughout human history. They will continue to draw on the energy and spiritual resources of those involved in the ministry of health care.

The healing services that we have attempted to describe in this chapter exist in many forms throughout the United States and the wider world. Some of the current searching for spiritual and physical healing emanates from the interest people have on the interplay between religion and health. Most of the mainline churches have included healing services in their regularly scheduled outreach to their parishioners. Not long ago, an Episcopal priest invited me to give a talk on prayer and healing for his congregation. The church was located in Flushing, Queens, New York. Services were conducted in three languages: English, Spanish, and Chinese. Interpreters are assigned for each of the three services. He had recently started these healing services. He remarked to me that he had been shocked to note that there were 267 people who showed up for the first of these services, each in search of physical, spiritual, and emotional help. This is only one small bit of evidence that churches need to reinforce their ministry of healing in order to represent to more people the providential healing power of God in their outreach to human suffering. Churches, in responding to people in such need, are also radiating the powerful compassionate presence of Jesus Christ and his Holy Spirit to those whose cries for healing are answered in ways as strange as the claims of Jesus that "the blind receive their sight, the lame walk, the lepers are cleansed, the deaf hear, the dead are raised, and the poor have good news brought to them" (Matthew 11:5).

DISCUSSION QUESTIONS

1. Comment on the statement in the Letter of James the Apostle that serves as the biblical basis for many healing services? Is this a practical directive?
2. Discuss the attitude of Ralph DiOrio toward the "wonders" effected in healing services.
3. Can we discuss the cases of Barbara MacRae and Alberto Barrera? How can we explain the miracles to which they attest?
4. What can we conclude from the story of Emily Gardiner Neal's conversion from skeptic to healing minister?
5. What lessons can we draw from the story of Susan's healing that took place in one of Father Ralph DiOrio's healing services?
6. How can we explain the phenomenon of some people being "cured" at healing services while others are just as sick afterward? Is it a question of faith?
7. Why is the laying on of hands so significant in healing services?
8. Comment on the claim that healing services can occur outside actual church buildings? Does location really matter when it is a question of the healing processes?
9. What is different about healing services conducted in locations as wide apart as a stadium and a prison? Comment on the value of such locations.
10. Why is it important to heal the whole person and not rest content with a physical betterment of a patient's condition? In what way can we say that responding to persons in need radiates the powerful compassionate presence of Jesus Christ?

Chapter 10

Conclusion: Health Care in the Power of the Spirit

Health care is a ministry of many dimensions, not least of which is its embeddedness in the power of God's Holy Spirit. In the biblical sense the Holy Spirit has been acknowledged as the divine creative force in Genesis bringing order out of chaos and life where none existed before. The Holy Spirit is the inspiration of the prophets, empowering them to criticize a nation that neglects its poor and forgotten. God's Spirit is the divine love energizing countless people of faith, who have been engaged in the healing of society's ills. To confess the role of faith and prayer in health care is not to denigrate the achievements of the scientific community in the practice of medicine. Nor is it a lessening of admiration for the technological advances that have enabled clinicians to overcome the stubborn causes of many diseases once thought to be both untreatable and incurable.

This book is not about substituting faith, prayer, and a spiritual relationship with God for the ministrations of capable health caregivers and the treatments available in today's well-equipped hospitals and clinics. To suggest, as we do, that health care is accomplished through power of the Spirit is to profess that, at the core of all the achievements of modern medicine and all the technological breakthroughs in health care, there lies the mysterious, often hidden, power of God.

HEALTH CARE EMPOWERED BY THE HOLY SPIRIT

We believe that the Holy Spirit of God permeates, indeed, makes possible the compassion and human creativity that have produced the so-called modern medical miracles and helped bring about a "better

Is There a God in Health Care?
© 2006 by The Haworth Press, Inc. All rights reserved.
doi:10.1300/5554_10

world." We also firmly believe that the healing process involves much more than the scientific, technological achievements, however effective these are in combating disease and illness. We have insisted here that God also acts through the spiritual life of health care providers and through ministries of healing in ways that are often directly related to the inner peace that has become a welcome adjunct to the practice of medicine. The act of praying with and for one's patients, for example, appears to have a either a direct or indirect effect on how patients may themselves be disposed to become involved in their own healing. The relationship of the health care provider to the patient can only be enhanced when the relationship is one of love, compassionate care, and intercessory prayer. At times, the healing that follows may seem to be totally the end result of the prayers offered for one struck down by disease. Many miracles of healing transcend medical possibilities and physicians can only join their own wonder. Many health caregivers, people of faith and prayer themselves, continue to marvel at the positive effects of intercessory prayer, the laying on of hands, and healing services on those with no other hope than recourse to the spiritual.

STRENGTH IN WEAKNESS

We do not claim this more spiritual interpretation of how God's power is related to the skills of the healer in order to exalt the practitioners of health care above the level of "ordinary" human beings. In all this, God can work wonders through the least probable of people. The Lord does, indeed, inspire health care providers to undertake the various healing ministries to those in need, even though they may themselves be coping with their own human foibles, sinfulness, or feelings of inadequacy. The Bible assures us that the Lord loves us just the way we are, the good in us along with the flaws. Despite our human weaknesses, we can be both healed by God and become, at the same time, channels for healing others. Dr. Daniel Sulmasy said it well:

> Holiness is not about being perfect. It is about the courage to acknowledge imperfection. It is about the courage to act in the face of imperfection. . . . It is the call to this kind of holiness that I want to urge upon health care professionals today. To be a

wounded healer is to be this kind of doctor or nurse. Holy, not by virtue of any saccharine practices or hypocritical pretensions of perfection. But holy by virtue of honesty. Holy by virtue of courage.[1]

Those Christians who work in the practice of health care are encouraged, not to mull over their obvious imperfections, but to see themselves engaged in a daring ministry of healing similar to that of Jesus.

The words of Saint Paul are a reminder that what God sees in people can be so different from our own limited vision:

> Consider your own call, brothers and sisters: not many of you were wise by human standards, not many were powerful, not many were of noble birth. But God chose what is foolish in the world to shame the wise; God chose what is weak in the world to shame the strong. (1 Corinthians 1:26-27)

Health care providers, conscious of their personal weaknesses, can only be encouraged by Paul's reassuring words. We also have Mark's supportive promise for Jesus' followers: "And these signs will accompany those who believe: . . . they will lay their hands on the sick, and they will recover" (Mark 16:17-18)—a salutary reminder that healing physical and spiritual ills is ultimately God's work.

Because the spiritual power of God radiates the healing of human ills at the mysterious center of health care, we believe it is important for those involved in this ministry to be more and more conscious of the blessedness of their calling. At the core of our communion with the divine is the Holy Spirit who creates in us the likeness and image of God, energizing our own spirit to take up the healing ministry.

AFFIRMING THE GOODNESS OF GOD
IN HEALTH CARE

The act of offering comfort to those crushed by their personal suffering is, in essence, a Spirit-driven, Christ-like undertaking in the ministry of health care. The Holy Spirit helps the health caregiver to see even the most destitute and physically repulsive with the eyes and compassionate attitude of our merciful, caring God. Given this vision, Jesuit Father Walter J. Burghardt called the Holy Spirit "the most dynamic force in the shaping of history."[2] Burghardt's fellow Jesuit Karl Rahner is equally insistent that the Holy Spirit is the dynamic link between the Trinitarian God and God's outgoing graciousness to us, God's children. The Holy Spirit can bring health care providers into an intercommunion with the divine source of their faith and ministry.

In attempting to discern how persons of faith can recognize and affirm God as Holy Spirit present in their profession, Rahner points out the signs.

> Wherever there is selfless love, wherever duties are carried out without hope of reward, wherever the incomprehensibility of death is calmly accepted, wherever people are good with no hope of reward; in all these instances the Spirit is experienced, even though a person may not dare give this interpretation to the experience.[3]

In Rahner's theology people are continually graced by the spirit of God's love from the moment of their coming into being and, certainly, even before they can say at all the name of Jesus in a faith commitment. Rahner appeals for boldness in listening to God's spirit and greater self-confidence in permitting one's entire self to be consumed by the "fire and energy of the Spirit." He urges believers not to stifle this Spirit but, permitting themselves to be led by God's Spirit, to become better persons able to shape society in the image of God from whom all creation has its meaning.

Rahner's perceptive acclamation of the work of the Holy Spirit, with all its implications for the ministry of health care, is not unlike the poetic exaltation of the Holy Spirit by Frederick Buechner. Buechner writes that, "to speak of the Holy Spirit is to speak above all . . . of the power of God, intoxicating, dangerous, world-transforming, irresistible." He cites Jesus' words to Nicodemus that the Holy Spirit acting in our lives is both "mysterious and unpredictable as the wind" (John 3:8).[4]

To be born by the wind of the Spirit? Could Jesus be saying that the workings of the Holy Spirit are so clandestine, so breathtaking, and so ungovernable that we are in the power of that Spirit without our even knowing it? The actions of the Holy Spirit are, indeed, mysterious to behold. We have affirmed in our common faith that the Holy Spirit moves us to break out of the stifling air of a stale routine. The

Holy Spirit is the creative force bestowing new vistas in the various ministries that comprise today's health care. When we are led by God's Spirit, our ways of thinking about people, events, and things of nature are changed. We become convinced that our life as God's children is stronger than sickness and even death and that new beginnings to physical, spiritual, and emotional health are possible where, before, one may have run into only dead ends where hope seemed to wither. The Holy Spirit continues to be the exciting soul of today's ministry of health care.

Keeping this in mind, we desired from the outset to speak of God, to whom we have dedicated our lives, as a God of compassion whose joy is to be present with us and whose sorrows are our sorrows. Time and again, we have professed our conviction that this is a God who suffers with us and cares for us as only a providential God can. This same God respects our freedom and does not violate the inexorable laws of our nature. This is a God who calls us to be the divine answer to those who cry out to God for deliverance from their sufferings and the pain that this chaotic world has caused.

We have written this book as a testament to our love of and gratitude to the ministry of healing and as an expression of our faith in the power of God at work in those who are called to care for those who suffer from physical, spiritual, and emotional ills in this imperfect world of ours. Both of us have been ourselves in need of the healing ministrations of others. We have been healed through the compassion of the many caring people who entered our lives in our times of need. Both of us have felt ourselves drawn by the power of the Spirit to undertake a ministry of healing, whether through the practice of medicine or in the teaching profession. We have benefited by the divine interventions in our moments of personal crises and brokenness. Early on in organizing our reflections, we decided to avoid rehashing analytical theories on suffering. Instead, we chose to share our personal stories with our readers in the hope that those involved in the ministry of health care can be strengthened in their own personal faith and, perhaps, come to a deeper appreciation of the role that God plays in every act of healing. We realize that many of our statements in this book are born out of the sufferings and joys that we have experienced and the influence so many others have had on our own healing. We draw, too, from the help we have been enabled to extend to those many others who have become part of our lives and shaped our understanding of the God who cares for us through Jesus and their spirit of love.

Many of our conclusions are traceable, not to empirical analysis, but to the faith with which God has endowed us. One day our faith will be transformed into the vision of God that is resurrection, and we will appreciate more fully the guidance of God seen in all the gentle ways in which we have been led to do God's work. In all our doubts, we take comfort in the words of Paul Tournier, the Swiss psychiatrist, who was himself touched by a sense of God's presence in his life.

> God guides us despite our uncertainties, and our vagueness, even through our failings and mistakes . . . Only afterwards, as we look back over the way we have come and reconsider certain important moments in our lives in the light of all that has followed them, or when we survey the whole progress of our lives do we experience the feeling of having been led without knowing it, the feeling that God has mysteriously guided us.[5]

Ultimately, the ministry of health care is under that mysterious guidance of God. This is especially true when a health care provider is on call, even in the middle of the night, and "hears" that "inner voice of God" urging him or her to get up and go to that patient, if only to be certain of what is going on. Examples abound of how patients' lives have been saved by the unexpected intervention of a health care provider who had listened to those mysterious promptings from what we, in faith, would call the inner voice of God's Spirit.

Finally, in this interim period in which we all live, whether in good or precarious health, and in the Spirit of Jesus Christ's Beatitudes, we offer the following.

Beatitudes for the Ministry of Health Care

1. Blessed are the health caregivers who will pray with and for their patients when they are hurting.
2. Blessed are the health caregivers who will help with quality care those of their patients who are poor and needy.

3. Blessed are the health caregivers who listen from the heart as their patients pour out their troubles.

4. Blessed are the health caregivers who are honest as well as gentle in communicating the truth of a patient's failing health.

5. Blessed are the health caregivers who are humble enough to admit their doubts and uncertainties when a patient's condition is difficult to diagnose.

6. Blessed are the health caregivers who, during their bedside visits, are compassionate and offer loving care when their patients are lonely, depressed, or confused.

7. Blessed are the health caregivers who palliate pain with their kind words, prayers, and supportive presence during their patients' dying days.

8. Blessed are the health caregivers who offer comfort and sympathy to the families of patients who have crossed the threshold of death into everlasting life.

In reflecting on the ministry of health caregivers as we have, we would be remiss if we neglected to acknowledge the recipients of their ministrations. Hence to them we offer this final Beatitude:

9. Blessed are those patients and individuals who put their trust in those who minister health care, whose courage, joys, and sorrows continue to be a neverending source of humility and inspiration.

DISCUSSION QUESTIONS

1. Comment on the assertion that the Holy Spirit makes possible the compassion and human creativity that have produced the so-called modern medical miracles and helped bring about a "better world."

2. What are the implications of the statement by Doctor Daniel Sulmasy on pp. 196-197?

3. What conclusions can be drawn from Mark's citation of Jesus' promise to his followers: "And these signs will accompany those

who believe: they will lay their hands on the sick, and they will recover" (Mark 16:17-18)?

4. Is it possible for health care providers to view their call as the
   divine answer to those who cry out to God for deliverance from
   their sufferings and the pain that this chaotic world has caused?
5. Discuss the Beatitudes for the Ministry of Health Care. Which are
   the most important? Why?

Notes

Chapter 1

1. These stories can be found in William F. Haynes Jr., *A Physician's Witness to the Power of Shared Prayer* (Chicago: Loyola University Press, 1990), 44-45, 51-52.

2. Abigail Zugar, "Are Doctors Losing Touch with Hands-on Medicine?" *The New York Times,* July 13, 1999, F1.

3. George Gallup and Andrew Greeley, *Newsweek,* March 20-21, 1997. This was a survey done by the Princeton Survey Research Associates, based on telephoning 751 adults nationwide.

4. "Caregiver," *Daily Word,* January 9, 1999.

5. Dietrich Bonhoeffer, *Letters and Papers from Prison* (New York: Macmillan, 1971), 361.

6. See Alexis Carrel, *Journey to Lourdes* (London: Hamish Hamilton, 1950).

7. See Albert Nolan, *Jesus Before Christianity* (Maryknoll: Orbis Press, 2001), 49.

8. See Saint Augustine, *The Confessions*, Volume III (New York: Vintage Spiritual Classics, 1998), 44.

9. Chuck Swindoll, *Growing Strong in the Seasons of Life* (Portland, OR: Multnomah Press, 1983), 238.

10. Haynes, *A Physician's Witness,* 29-31.

11. See William F. Haynes, *Minding the Whole Person: Cultivating a Healthy Lifestyle from Youth through the Senior Years* (Chicago: Loyola University Press, 1994).

Chapter 2

1. Randolph C. Byrd, "Positive Therapeutic Effects of Intercessory Prayer in a Coronary Care Unit Population," *Southern Medical Journal,* 81, 7 (1989), 826-829.

2. Jeremy D. Kark, "Does Religious Observance Promote Health? Mortality in Secular vs. Religious Kibbutzim in Israel," *American Journal of Public Health,* 86 (1996), 341-346.

3. Phyllis McIntosh, "Faith Is Powerful Medicine," *Remedy,* Nov./Dec. (1997), 29.

4. Ralph DiOrio, *The Healing Power of Affirmation: Accepting God and Goodness in Your Life* (New York: Doubleday Image Book, 1985), 99.

5. Francis MacNutt, *Healing* (Notre Dame: Ave Maria Press, 1975), 132.

Is There a God in Health Care?
© 2006 by The Haworth Press, Inc. All rights reserved.
doi:10.1300/5554_11

6. See Saint Augustine, *The Confessions,* Volume III (New York: Vintage Spiritual Classics, 1998), 44.

7. Søren Kierkegaard, *Philosophical Fragments,* 4, 254.

8. Louis Dupré, *Kierkegaard As Theologian* (New York: Sheed & Ward, 1963), 128-129.

9. See Paul Tillich, *Dynamics of Faith* (New York: Harper Torchback, 1958).

10. Dietrich Bonhoeffer, *Ethics* (New York: Macmillan, 1965), 243-244.

11. Dietrich Bonhoeffer, *Letters and Papers from Prison* (New York: Macmillan, 1971), 14.

12. Ibid., 369.

13. Ibid., 382.

14. Dietrich Bonhoeffer, *Discipleship,* John D. Godsey and Geffrey B. Kelly, eds. (Minneapolis: Fortress Press, 2000), 87.

15. Karl Rahner, *The Great Church Year: The Best of Karl Rahner's Homilies, Sermons and Meditations* (New York: Crossroad, 1995), 319.

16. Eugene Kennedy, *Believing* (New York: Doubleday, 1974), 17.

17. Ernest Gordon, *Through the Valley of the Kwai: From Death-Camp Despair to Spiritual Triumph* (New York: Harper and Brothers, 1962), 52.

18. Ibid., 113.

19. Ibid., 137.

20. Ibid., 255.

21. Joseph Cardinal Bernardin, *The Gift of Peace* (New York: Doubleday Image Book, 1997), 6-7.

22. See "Bernardin," Martin Doblmeier, Director, Journey/Frost Productions and Family Theatre Productions in association with Santa Fe Communications, 1998.

23. Cited in William O'Brien, "Vanier: Called to Compassion," *The Other Side,* March 1986, 16.

24. Ibid., 15.

25. Ibid., 17; see also "The Heart Has Its Reasons," Martin Doblmeier, Director, Journey Communications, 1984.

26. Ibid., 21.

27. Gordon Mursell, "Mother Teresa of Calcutta (1910-97)," *The Story of Christian Spirituality* (Minneapolis: Fortress Press, 2001), 322.

28. Mother Teresa, *A Gift for God: Prayers and Meditations* (San Francisco: HarperCollins Publishers, Inc., 1975), 74.

29. Mursell, *The Story of Christian Spirituality,* 322.

30. Kennedy, *Believing,* 120.

Chapter 3

1. Thomas à Kempis, *The Imitation of Christ* (Garden City, NY: Doubleday, 1962), 32.

2. Luke Salm, *The Work Is Yours: The Life of Soul John Baptist de La Salle* (Landover, MD: Christian Brothers Publications, 1996), 188.

3. Martin Luther, "Vorrede zur Neuburger Psalterausgabe," 1545, *Deutsche Bibel, WA,* 10/2: 157.

4. Walter Bruggemann, "A Case Study in Daring Prayer," *The Living Pulpit,* Vol. 2, No. 3 (July-September, 1993), 12-13.

5. Ann Hallstein, "Presence As Prayer," *The Living Pulpit,* Vol. 2, No. 3 (July-September, 1993), 38-39.

6. Ibid.

7. Dietrich Bonhoeffer in Geffrey B. Kelly and F. Burton Nelson, eds., *A Testament to Freedom: The Essential Writings of Dietrich Bonhoeffer* (San Francisco: HarperCollins, 1995), 457.

8. Gloria Hutchinson, *Six Ways to Pray from Six Great Saints* (Cincinnati, OH: St. Anthony Messenger Press, 1996), 112-118.

9. Dietrich Bonhoeffer, *Life Together,* Geffrey B. Kelly, ed. (Minneapolis: Fortress Press, 1995), 90.

10. Dietrich Bonhoeffer, *Letters and Papers from Prison* (New York: Macmillan, 1971), 131.

11. Karl Rahner, "Who Are Your Brother and Sister?" In Geffrey B. Kelly, ed., *Karl Rahner: Theologian of the Graced Search for Meaning* (Minneapolis: Fortress Press, 1992), 319.

12. Bonhoefer, in *A Testament to Freedom,* 59.

13. Brother Lawrence of the Resurrection, *The Practice of the Presence of God* (Springfield, IL: Templegate Publisher, 1974).

14. David H.C. Read, "So You're Preaching on Prayer? God Help You," *The Living Pulpit,* Vol. 2, No. 3 (July-September, 1993), 11.

15. Miriam Murphy, *Prayer in Action: A Growth Experience* (Nashville: Abingdon, 1979), 43.

16. William F. Haynes, *A Physician's Witness to the Power of Shared Prayer* (Chicago: Loyola University Press, 1990), 2-6.

Chapter 4

1. Dietrich Bonhoeffer, *Letters and Papers from Prison* (New York: Macmillan, 1971), 360-361; translation slightly altered.

2. Dietrich Bonhoeffer, *Life Together,* Geffrey B. Kelly, ed. (Minneapolis: Fortress Press, 1995), 99.

3. The NRSV translates Mark 14:33-35 as "[He] began to be distressed and agitated. And he said to them, 'I am deeply grieved, even to death . . .'"

4. Daniel P. Sulmasy, *The Healers' Calling: A Spirituality for Physicians and Other Health Care Professions* (New York: Paulist Press, 1997), 108.

5. Ibid.

6. See also the book on which the film was based, Sylvia Nasor, *A Beautiful Mind* (New York: Simon & Schuster Touchstone Book, 1998).

7. See Michael J. Fox, *Lucky Man: A Memoir* (New York: Hyperion Press, 2002).

8. Sermon by Reverend Jay Sibebotham, St. Bartholomew's Church, New York, February 10, 2002.

9. Lyndon Harris, "It's Easter at Ground Zero," *Episcopal Life,* April 2002, 17, 22.

10. Robert Stern, "Widow's Solace Was Her Faith," *Trenton Times*, March 27, 2002, A1.

11. Daniel Lewis, "Mister Rogers, TV's Friend for Children, Is Dead at 74," *The New York Times*, February 28, 2003, A1, B11.

Chapter 5

1. Philip Simmons, *Learning to Fall: The Blessings of an Imperfect Life* (New York: Bantam Books, 2001).

2. James R. Kok, *Waiting for Morning: Seeking God in Our Suffering* (Grand Rapids: CRC Publications, 1997), 112.

3. Bruce Chilton, "Suffering in the Light of the Gospel," *The Living Pulpit*, 4, 2 (April-June 1995), 25.

4. Walter J. Burghardt, "Suffering: Aging and Dying," *The Living Pulpit*, 4, 2 (April-June 1995), 7.

5. Ibid.

6. Matthew Fox, *A Spirituality Named Compassion & The Healing of the Global Village* (Minneapolis: Winston Press, 1979), 33.

7. Ibid., 34.

8. Kenneth Ring, *Heading Toward Omega: In Search of the Meaning of the Near-Death Experience* (New York: William Morrow and Company, 1985).

9. Ibid., see the section "Core NDEs: Some Illustrative Cases," 53ff.

10. George Maloney, *Death, Where Is Your Sting?* (New York: Alba House, 1984), 13.

11. H. Norman Wright, *Recovering from the Losses of Life* (Grand Rapids: Baker Revell Books, 2000).

12. Evelyn Underhill, *Mysticism* (New York: Doubleday, 1990), 20.

13. John Calvin, *On the Christian Life*, cited by John S. Mogabgab in his "Editor's Introduction," to the special issue on Suffering, *Weavings*, 17, 5 (September/October 2002), 3.

14. Robert C. Morris, "Suffering and the Courage of God," *Weavings*, 17, 5 (October 2002), 9.

15. Ibid., 12-13.

16. Dietrich Bonhoeffer, *Letters and Papers from Prison* (New York: Macmillan, 1971), 14.

17. See Henri Nouwen, *The Wounded Healer: Ministry in Contemporary Society* (Garden City: Doubleday, 1972).

18. Ginger Grab, "Shakespeare's King Lear: Gaining a Soul," *The Living Pulpit*, 4, 2 (April-June 1995), 23.

19. Harold S. Kushner, *When Bad Things Happen to Good People* (New York: Avon Books, 1981), 110-111.

20. David Rensberger, "Suffering Together Before God," *Weavings*, 17, 5 (September/October 2002), 43.

21. Kushner, *When Bad Things Happen to Good People*, 129.

22. Ibid., 31-45.

23. Ibid., 140.

24. Ibid., 148.

25. J. Gerald Janzen, "Walking Through the Valley of the Shadow of Death," *The Living Pulpit*, 7, 3 (July-September 1998), 23.

26. Karl Rahner, cited by Janzen in Ibid., 23.

27. Karl Rahner, cited in Geffrey B. Kelly, *Karl Rahner: Theologian of the Graced Search for Meaning* (Minneapolis: Fortress Press, 1992), 31.

28. Karl Rahner, *Theological Investigations* (New York: Crossroads, 1974), 391.

29. Karl Rahner, *Foundations of Christian Faith* (New York: Seabury Press, 1978), 143.

30. Mitch Album, *Tuesdays with Morrie: An Old Man, a Young Man, and Life's Greatest Lesson* (New York: Doubleday, 1997), 57.

31. Natalie Babbitt, *Tuck Everlasting* (New York: Farrar, Straus and Giroux, 2002), 63-64.

32. Album, *Tuesdays with Morrie*, 35-36.

33. "Bernardin," Martin Doblmeier, Director, Journey/Frost Productions and Family Theater Productions in association with Santa Fe Communications, 1998.

34. Joseph Cardinal Bernardin, *The Gift of Peace* (New York: Doubleday Image Books, 1997), 92.

35. Ibid., 126.

36. Ibid., xiii.

37. Bonhoeffer, *Letters and Papers from Prison*, 391.

Chapter 6

1. Dietrich Bonhoeffer, *Letters and Papers from Prison* (New York: Macmillan, 1971), 46.

2. Michael Buckley, *His Healing Touch* (London: Font Paperbacks, 1997), 1.

3. Paul Tournier, *Reflections* (Philadelphia: The Westminster Press, 1976), 69.

4. Brother Roger of Taizé, *Parable of Community* (Oxford, UK: A.R. Mowbray and Co., 1984), p. 78.

5. Brother Roger of Taizé, *Life from Within* (Louisville: Westminster/John Knox, 1990), 28.

6. Henri Nouwen, *Life of the Beloved: Spiritual Living in a Secular World* (New York: Crossroad, 1993), 27.

7. Ibid., 88.

8. Gary Ross, "Moving Beyond Blame," *The New York Times,* May 6, 1999, A33.

9. Barbara L. Shlemon, *Healing Power* (Notre Dame: Ave Maria Press, 1982), 27.

10. Eddie Ensley, *Prayer That Heals Our Emotions* (Columbus, GA: Contemplative Books, 1986), 61.

11. Daniel Sulmasy, *The Healer's Calling* (New York: Paulist Press, 1997), 14.

12. Agnes Sanford, *The Healing Gifts of the Spirit* (Philadelphia: Trumpet Books, 1966), 10.

13. Ibid., 29

14. Ibid., 30.

15. Barbara L. Shlemon, *Healing the Inner Self*, 10.

16. Jean Vanier, *The Broken Body: Journey to Wholeness* (Mahwah: Paulist Press, 1994), 69.

17. Dietrich Bonhoeffer, "Christ's Love and Our Enemies," Sermon, *A Testament to Freedom*, January 23, 1938, 287-288.

18. Daniel Day Williams, *The Spirit and the Forms of Love* (New York: Harper and Row, 1968), 5.

19. Ibid.

20. Ibid., 138.

21. Anna Freud, quoted in Robert Coles, *Dorothy Day: A Radical Devotion* (New York: Addison Wesley Publishing Company, 1987), 155.

22. Doris Donnelly, *Learning to Forgive* (New York: Macmillan Publishing Co., 1979), 19.

23. Martin Luther King Jr., *The Strength to Love* (New York: Pocket Books, 1964), 33.

24. Roger Lovette, "The Essence of the Gospel," *The Living Pulpit*, 3, 2 (April-June, 1994), 42.

25. Frederick Buechner, *Wishful Thinking: A Theological ABC* (New York: Harper and Row, 1973), 29.

26. Desmond Tutu, "Forgiveness and Reconciliation," *Home Page*, Church of the Holy Family, Chapel Hill, NC, October 5, 2001.

27. Ibid.

28. Ibid.

29. Corrie ten Boom, *The Hiding Place* (Old Tappan, NJ: Chosen Books, 1984), 214-215.

30. Henri Nouwen, cited in Donnelly, *Learning to Forgive*, 71.

31. Pope John Paul II, "Religions of the World in the Service of Peace," *The Pope Speaks*, 47, 5 (January 24, 2002), 269.

Chapter 7

1. Oliver Wendell Holmes, "Poet at the Breakfast Table," *Atlantic Monthly*, 1872, cited in the *Oxford Dictionary of Quotations* (Oxford and New York: Oxford University Press, 1992), 342.

2. This line is take from the hymn "The Cry of the Poor," based on Psalm 34:6. See hymn 523 from *Breaking Bread with Readings* (Portland, OR: Oregon Catholic Press, 2006).

3. Dietrich Bonhoeffer, *Life Together*, Geffrey B. Kelly, ed. (Minneapolis: Fortress Press, 1995), 98.

4. John Stott, *The Contemporary Christian: An Urgent Plea for Double Listening* (Leicester, UK: Inter-varsity Press, 1992), 13.

5. Bonhoeffer, *Life Together*, 98; emphasis ours.

6. Ibid., translation slightly altered.

7. Paul Tournier, *A Listening Ear: Reflections on Christian Caring* (Minneapolis: Augsburg Publishing House, 1987), 12.

8. Ibid., 140-141.

9. Frederick Buechner, *The Sacred Journey* (San Francisco: Harper and Row, 1982), 77-78.

10. William Tully, in a draft of the sermon preached on December 13, 1998, and sent by him to William F. Haynes.

11. Bishop Thomas Shaw, Lecture at Trinity Cathedral, Trenton, NJ, January 26, 2001, as recorded by William F. Haynes.

12. Anthony de Mello, *One Minute Wisdom* (Garden City, NY: Doubleday, 1986), 175.

13. Gerald Kamens, "Listening," *America,* 187, 15 (November 11, 2002), 22-23.

Chapter 8

1. Martin Luther King Jr., "A Time to Break Silence," in *I Have a Dream: Writings and Speeches That Changed the World,* James M. Washington, ed. (San Francisco: HarperCollins, 1992), 148.

2. See Dom Helder Camara, "Wisdom Quotes," in Dom Helder Camara: A Mystic in Love with the Poor. Available online at http://www.domhelder.com.br/ingles/politics.htm.

3. Quoted by Donald W. Shriver Jr., in "Suffering at Second Hand," *The Living Pulpit,* 4, 2 (April-June 1995), 14.

4. Ibid.

5. Dietrich Bonhoeffer, *Letters and Papers from Prison* (New York: Macmillan, 1971), 17.

6. See "Household Food Security in the United States, 2002," *ERS Research Briefs–USDA,* Government Publications, 2005.

7. "The Non-Paying Class," *Wall Street Journal,* November 20, 2002, Editorial page.

8. "One in Three: Non-Elderly Americans Without Health Insurance, 2002-2003," *Families USA,* Government Publications, 2005.

9. Jennifer Potash, "Beware Orwellian 'efficiency,' Reinhardt cautions, Health economist ridicules views of his own profession," *Princeton Packet,* April 23, 1999, p. 3A.

10. Ibid.

11. Jean Vanier, *The Broken Body: Journey to Wholeness* (Mahwah, NJ: Paulist Press, 1994), 45.

12. Jurgen Moltmann, "The Destruction and Healing of the Earth," in Max L. Stackhouse and Don S. Browning, eds., *God and Globalization: The Spirit and the Modern Authorities,* Volume 2 (Harrisburg, PA: Trinity Press International, 2001), 168.

13. Todd Post, "Frontline Issues in Nutrition Assistance: Bread for the World Institute's 16th Annual Report on the State of World Hunger," Executive summary. Available online at http://www.bread.org/institute/hunger_report/2006_executive_summary.htm. Bread for the World Institute, 2005.

14. Stanford Recycling Center, "Recycling," available online at http://recycling.stanford.edu/5r/recycle.html, Peninsula Sanitary Service, Inc. 2000.

15. Satish Kenchaiah, Jane C. Evans, Daniel Levy, Peter W.F. Wilson, Emelia J. Benjamin, Martin G. Larson, William B. Kannel, and Ramachandran S. Vasan, "Obesity and the Risk of Heart Failure," *New England Journal of Medicine,* 347, 5 (August 2002), 305.

16. Sudarsan Raghavan, "From Man and Nature, Starvation," *The Philadelphia Inquirer Sunday Review,* January 26, 2003, C1. Emphasis added.

17. Ibid.

18. Ibid., C3.

19. John McDonald, United States Coordinator for the United Nations Decade on Drinking Water and Sanitation, 1980, www.Globalwater.org.

20. "Water for a Thirsty World," *The New York Times,* August 29, 2002, A24.

21. Alberto Múnera, "New Theology on Population, Ecology, and Overconsumption from the Catholic Perspective," in Harold Coward and Daniel C. Maguire, eds., *Visions of a New Earth: Religious Perspectives on Population, Consumption, and Ecology* (New York: SUNY Press, 2000), 66-67.

22. James A. Nash, *Loving Nature: Ecological Integrity and Christian Responsibility* (Nashville: Abingdon Press in Cooperation with the Churches' Center for Theology and Public Policy, 1991), 28.

23. Ibid., 32.

24. Ibid.

25. Rosemary Radford Ruether, "Global Capitalism: A New Challenge to Theologians," *National Catholic Reporter,* February 7, 2003, 16.

26. John MacArthur, *Second Front: Censorship and Propaganda in the Gulf War* (New York: Hill and Wang, 1992), 246-247.

27. Ibid., 35.

28. George J. Bryjak, "Don't Call It War—It's Mass Horror," *National Catholic Reporter,* February 7, 2003, 18.

29. Ibid.

30. Robert Drinan, "Bush's Unilateralism Aggravates World's Problems," *National Catholic Reporter,* January 10, 2003, 16.

31. Peter J. Paris, "Moral Exemplars in Global Community," in Max L. Stackhouse and Don S. Browning, eds., *God and Globalization: The Spirit and the Modern Authorities,* Volume 2 (Harrisburg, PA: Trinity Press International, 2001), 219.

Chapter 9

1. Ralph A. DiOrio, *Signs and Wonders: Firsthand Experiences of Healing* (New York: Doubleday Image Books, 1987), 14.

2. Ibid., 81-82.

3. Ibid.

4. Ibid.

5. Ibid., 83.

6. Ibid., 43.

7. Ibid., 45.

8. Emily Gardiner Neal, *A Reporter Finds God Through Spiritual Healing* (New York: Morehouse-Gorsham Co., 1956), 1-7.

9. Anne Cassel, ed., *Emily Gardiner Neal: Celebration of Healing* (Cambridge, MA: Cowley Publications, 1992), 1-11.

10. Ibid., 9.

11. Ibid., 10-11.

12. Personal communication from Father Orsini.

13. Francis MacNutt, *Healing* (Notre Dame: Ave Maria Press, 1975), 132.

14. Ibid.

15. Kathryn Kuhlman, cited in Ibid., 146.
16. Ibid., 147.

Chapter 10

1. Daniel Sulmasy, *The Healers' Calling: A Spirituality for Physicians and Other Health Care Professions* (New York: Paulist Press, 1997), 108, 123.

2. Walter J. Burghardt, "The Spirit Is Dynamite," *The Living Pulpit,* 5, 1 (January-March 1996), 5.

3. Cited in Geffrey B. Kelly, "The Everyday Experience of God: Karl Rahner's Theology of the Holy Spirit," *The Living Pulpit,* 5, 1 (January-March 1996), 35.

4. Frederick Buechner, "The Holy Spirit: The Power of God," *The Living Pulpit,* 5, 1 (January-March 1996), 14.

5. Paul Tournier, *Reflections* (Philadelphia: Westminster Press, 1976), 123.

Bibliography

Album, Mitch. *Tuesdays with Morrie: An Old Man, a Young Man, and Life's Greatest Lesson.* New York: Doubleday, 1997.

Augustine, Saint. *The Confessions.* New York: Vintage Spiritual Classics, 1998.

Babbit, Natalie. *Tuck Everlasting.* New York: Farrar, Straus and Giroux, 2002.

Bernardin, Joseph Cardinal. *The Gift of Peace.* New York: Doubleday Image Books, 1997.

Bonhoeffer, Dietrich. *Discipleship,* ed. by John D. Godsey and Geffrey B. Kelly. Minneapolis: Fortress Press, 2001.

Bonhoeffer, Dietrich. *Letters and Papers from Prison.* New York: Macmillan, 1971.

Bonhoeffer, Dietrich. *Life Together,* ed. by Geffrey B. Kelly. Minneapolis: Fortress Press, 1995.

Bonhoeffer, Dietrich. *A Testament to Freedom: The Essential Writings of Dietrich Bonhoeffer,* ed. by Geffrey B. Kelly and F. Burton Nelson. San Francisco: HarperCollins, 1995.

Brother Lawrence of the Resurrection. *The Practice of the Presence of God.* Springfield, IL: Templegate Publishers, 1974.

Browne, Elizabeth J. *The Disabled Disciple: Ministering in a Church Without Barriers.* Liguori, MO: Libuori Publications, 1997.

Buechner, Frederick. *Listening to Your Life: Daily Meditations.* San Francisco: HarperCollins, 1992.

Close, Henry. *Becoming a Forgiving Person: A Pastoral Perspective.* Binghamton, NY: The Haworth Press, 2004.

Coles, Robert. *Dorothy Day: A Radical Devotion.* New York: Addison Wesley Publishing Company, 1987.

Daily Word. January 9, 1999. Unity Village, MO: Unity.

De Mello, Anthony. *One Minute Wisdom.* Garden City, NY: Doubelday, 1986.

De Vinck, Christopher. *The Power of the Powerless.* Grand Rapids, MI: Zondervan, 1995.

DiOrio, Fr. Ralph A. *Signs and Wonders: Firsthand Experiences of Healing.* Garden City, NY: Doubleday Image Books, 1971.

DiOrio, Fr. Ralph A. *The Healing Power of Affirmation: Accepting God and Goodness in Your Life.* Garden City: Doubleday Image Books, 1986.

DiOrio, Fr. Ralph A. *Healing Love: A Treasury of Healing Prayers and Blessings to Help You Through Life's Hurts.* New York: Doubleday, 1988.

Is There a God in Health Care?
© 2006 by The Haworth Press, Inc. All rights reserved.
doi:10.1300/5554_12

Donnelly, Doris. *Learning to Forgive.* New York: Macmillan Publishing Co., 1979.

Dossey, Larry. *Recovering the Soul: A Scientific and Spiritual Search.* New York: Doubleday Bantam Books, 1989.

Ensley, Eddie. *Prayer That Heals Our Emotions.* Columbus, GA: Contemplative Books, 1986.

Evans, Abigail R. *Redeeming Marketplace Medicine: A Theology of Health Care.* Cleveland: The Pilgrim Press, 1999.

Fox, Matthew. *A Spirituality Named Compassion & the Healing of the Global Village.* Minneapolis: Winston Press, 1979.

Gordon, Ernest. *Through the Valley of the Kwai: From Death-Camp Despair to Spiritual Triumph.* New York: Harper and Brothers, 1962.

Haynes, William F. *A Physician's Witness to the Power of Shared Prayer.* Chicago: Loyola University Press, 1990.

Haynes, William F. *Minding the Whole Person: Cultivating a Healthy Lifestyle from Youth Through the Senior Years.* Chicago: Loyola University Press, 1994.

Hildegard of Bingen. *Holistic Healing.* Collegeville, MN: Liturgical Press, 1994.

Hutchinson, Gloria. *Six Ways to Pray from Six Great Saints.* Cincinnati, OH: St. Anthony Messenger Press, 1996.

Johnson, Timothy. *Find God in the Questions: A Personal Journey.* Downer's Grove, IL: InterVarsity Press, 2004.

Kahle, Peter and John M. Robbins. *The Power of Spirituality in Therapy: Integrating Spiritual and Religious Beliefs in Mental Health Practice.* Binghamton, NY: The Haworth Press, 2004.

Kelly, David F. *Critical Care Ethics: Treatment Decisions in American Hospitals.* Lanham, MD: Sheed & Ward, 1991.

Kennedy, Eugene. *Believing.* New York: Doubleday, 1974.

King, Dana E. *Faith, Spirituality, and Medicine: Toward the Making of a Healing Practitioner.* Binghamton, NY: The Haworth Press, 2000.

Koenig, Harold G. *Aging and God: Spiritual Pathways to Mental Health in Midlife and Later Years.* Binghamton, NY: The Haworth Press, 1994.

Koenig, Harold G. *Chronic Pain: Biomedical and Spiritual Approaches.* Binghamton, NY: The Haworth Press, 2002.

Koenig, Harold G. *Spirituality in Patient Care: Why, How, When, and What.* Philadelphia: Templeton Foundation Press, 2002.

Kübler-Ross, Elisabeth. *The Wheel of Life: A Memoir of Living and Dying.* New York: Simon and Schuster, 1997.

Kuhlman, Kathryn. *I Believe in Miracles.* North Brunswick, NJ: Bridge-Logos Publishers, 1990.

Kushner, Harold S. *When Bad Things Happen to Good People.* New York: Avon Books, 1983.

Levine, Stephen. *Healing into Life and Death.* New York: Doubleday Anchor Books, 1987.

MacArthur, John. *Second Front: Censorship and Propaganda in the Gulf War.* New York: Hill and Wang, 1992.

MacNutt, Francis. *Healing.* Notre Dame: Ave Maria Press, 1975.

MacNutt, Francis. *The Power to Heal.* Notre Dame: Ave Maria Press, 1977.

McCall, Junietta Baker. *Bereavement Counseling: Pastoral Care for Complicated Grieving.* Binghamton, NY: The Haworth Press, 2004.

Mohrmann, Margaret E. and Mark J. Hanson, eds. *Pain Seeking Understanding.* Cleveland: The Pilgrim Press, 1999.

Murphy, Miriam. *Prayer in Action: A Growth Experience.* Nashville: Abingdon, 1979.

Mursell, Gordon. *The Story of Christian Spirituality.* Minneapolis: Fortress Press, 2001.

Neal, Emily Gardiner. *Celebration of Healing,* ed. by Barbara Shlemon. Cambridge, MA: Cowley Publications, 1992.

Nouwen, Henri. *The Wounded Healer: Ministry in Contemporary Society.* Garden City, NY: Doubleday, 1972.

Nouwen, Henri. *Adam: God's Beloved.* Maryknoll, NY: Orbis Books, 1997.

Ring, Kenneth. *Heading Toward Omega: In Search of the Meaning of the Near-Death Experience.* New York: William Morrow and Co., 1985.

Russell, Keith A, Editor. "Healing," Special Issue of *The Living Pulpit,* Vol. 6, No. 2 (April-June 1997).

Salm, Luke. *The Work Is Yours: The Life of Saint John Baptist de La Salle,* Landover, MD: Christian Brothers Publications, 1996.

Stearn, Jess. *Edgar Cayce: The Sleeping Prophet.* New York: Bantam Books, 1968.

Sulmasy, Daniel P. *The Healer's Calling: A Spirituality for Physicians and Other Health Care Professions.* New York: Paulist Press, 1997.

Tada, Joni Eareckson. *The God I Love.* Grand Rapids, MI: Zondervan, 2003.

Ten Boom, Corrie, with John and Elizabeth Sherrill. *The Hiding Place.* Grand Rapids: Chosen Books, 1984.

Thomas à Kempis. *The Imitation of Christ,* edited by Harold C. Gardiner. Garden City, NY: Doubelday, 1962.

Tolson, Chester L. and Harold G. Koenig. *Healing Power of Prayer: The Surprising Connection Between Prayer and Your Health.* Grand Rapids: Baker Books, 2004.

Vanier, Jean. *The Broken Body: Journey to Wholeness.* New York: Paulist Press, 1994.

Vanier, Jean. *Our Journey Home: Rediscovering a Common Humanity Beyond Our Differences.* Maryknoll, NY: Orbis, 1997.

Walters, Jack. *Jesus: Healer of Our Inner World.* New York: Crossroad, 1996.

Wuellner, Flora Slosson. *Forgiveness, the Passionate Journey: Nine Steps of Forgiving Through Jesus' Beatitudes.* Nashville: Upper Room Books, 2001.

Index

AIDS (Acquired Immune Deficiency Syndrome), 163,164,188
Album, Mitch, 114, 207, 213
Allen, Woody, 113
ALS (Amyotrophic Lateral Sclerosis-Lou Gehrig's Disease), 94
Anointing, 175-176
Augustine, 10, 24, 203, 213

Babbitt, Natalie, 207, 213
Barrera, Albert, 178-179, 194
Beamer, Lisa, 88-89
Bernardin, Joseph Cardinal, 33-34, 117, 118, 204, 207
Bethge, Eberhard, 28, 52, 117
Bilhuber, Ernest, 61
Biotechnology, 2, 3
Bonaventure, *x, xi, xiv*
Bonding, 2, 39
Bonhoeffer, Dietrich, *x-xiv*, 6, 27-29, 36, 40, 50, 52, 53-54, 69-70, 74, 107, 114, 117-118, 119-120, 129-130, 137, 139-140, 144, 158, 173, 203, 204, 205, 206, 207, 208, 209, 213
Brokenness
  in divorce, 62
  dying to self, 95, 100
  perseverance, 30
  and spirituality, 83-84
  unexpected loss, 59
Brother André, 185
Brother Lawrence, 58, 205, 213
Browne, Elizabeth, 213
Bruggemann, Walter, 48, 204

Bryjak, George, 169, 210
Buckley, Michael, 20, 207
Buechner, Frederick, 133, 145-146, 154, 198, 208, 211, 213
Bultmann, Rudolf, *x*
Burghardt, Walter, 95, 197-198, 206, 211
Bush, George W., 164
Byrd, Randolph, 21, 203

Calvin, John, 206
Camara, Dom Helder, 156, 209
Carmody, Sister M.L., 64
Carrel, Alexis, 7, 203
Carter, Jimmy, 171
Cassell, Anne, 210
CCU, Coronary Care Unit, 16, 86, 87
Charismatic healing, 63, 176-179, 190
Chemotherapy, 79-80, 81, 105, 117, 181
Chesterton, Gilbert Keith, 87
Chilton, Bruce, 95, 206
Close, Henry, 213
Coles, Robert, 213
Collateral damage, 169
Columbine massacre, 125
Community
  availability for others, 74
  of believers, 124
  in giving love, 125
  in listening as service, 100-102, 140
  reaching out, 126-127
  in suffering, 99-104
Compassion
  in community, 125
  consolation in grief, 99-100

Is There a God in Health Care?
© 2006 by The Haworth Press, Inc. All rights reserved.
doi:10.1300/5554_13

Order a copy of this book with this form or online at:
http://www.haworthpress.com/store/product.asp?sku=5554

IS THERE A GOD IN HEALTH CARE?
Toward a New Spirituality of Medicine

_____in hardbound at $39.95 (ISBN-13: 978-0-7890-2866-2; ISBN-10: 0-7890-2866-2)

_____in softbound at $24.95 (ISBN-13: 978-0-7890-2867-9; ISBN-10: 0-7890-2867-0)

Or order online and use special offer code HEC25 in the shopping cart.

COST OF BOOKS_____

☐ **BILL ME LATER:** (Bill-me option is good on US/Canada/Mexico orders only; not good to jobbers, wholesalers, or subscription agencies.)

☐ Check here if billing address is different from shipping address and attach purchase order and billing address information.

POSTAGE & HANDLING_____
(US: $4.00 for first book & $1.50 for each additional book)
(Outside US: $5.00 for first book & $2.00 for each additional book)

Signature_____

SUBTOTAL_____

☐ **PAYMENT ENCLOSED: $**_____

IN CANADA: ADD 7% GST_____

☐ **PLEASE CHARGE TO MY CREDIT CARD.**

STATE TAX_____
(NJ, NY, OH, MN, CA, IL, IN, PA, & SD residents, add appropriate local sales tax)

☐ Visa ☐ MasterCard ☐ AmEx ☐ Discover
☐ Diner's Club ☐ Eurocard ☐ JCB

Account # _____

FINAL TOTAL_____
(If paying in Canadian funds, convert using the current exchange rate, UNESCO coupons welcome)

Exp. Date_____

Signature_____

Prices in US dollars and subject to change without notice.

NAME_____

INSTITUTION_____

ADDRESS_____

CITY_____

STATE/ZIP_____

COUNTRY_____ COUNTY (NY residents only)_____

TEL_____ FAX_____

E-MAIL_____

May we use your e-mail address for confirmations and other types of information? ☐ Yes ☐ No We appreciate receiving your e-mail address and fax number. Haworth would like to e-mail or fax special discount offers to you, as a preferred customer. **We will never share, rent, or exchange your e-mail address or fax number.** We regard such actions as an invasion of your privacy.

Order From Your Local Bookstore or Directly From
The Haworth Press, Inc.
10 Alice Street, Binghamton, New York 13904-1580 • USA
TELEPHONE: 1-800-HAWORTH (1-800-429-6784) / Outside US/Canada: (607) 722-5857
FAX: 1-800-895-0582 / Outside US/Canada: (607) 771-0012
E-mail to: orders@haworthpress.com

For orders outside US and Canada, you may wish to order through your local
sales representative, distributor, or bookseller.
For information, see http://haworthpress.com/distributors

(Discounts are available for individual orders in US and Canada only, not booksellers/distributors.)

PLEASE PHOTOCOPY THIS FORM FOR YOUR PERSONAL USE.
http://www.HaworthPress.com   BOF06